Sweat. Eat. Repeat.

The 90-day playbook to change your food habits, improve your energy, and reach your goals

Pamela Nisevich Bede
MS, RD, CSSD, LD

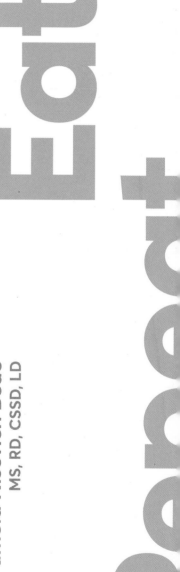

VELO
press

Boulder, Colorado

*To Miller, Hunter, and Piper: May you be brave enough to
march to the beat of your own drum, fit enough to race to the
front of the pack, kind enough to care for the welfare of others,
and may you always remember that you are my number one.*

4745 Walnut Street, Unit A
Boulder, CO 80301–2587 USA

VeloPress is the leading publisher of books on endurance sports and is a division
of Pocket Outdoor Media. Focused on cycling, triathlon, running, swimming, and
nutrition/diet, VeloPress books help athletes achieve their goals of going faster
and farther. Preview books and contact us at velopress.com.

Distributed in the United States and Canada by Ingram Publisher Services

A Cataloging-in-Publication record for this book is available from the
Library of Congress. ISBN 978-1-948007-00-9

This paper meets the requirements of ANSI/NISO Z39.48-1992
(Permanence of Paper).

Art direction by Vicki Hopewell
Design by Kevin Roberson

19 20 21 / 10 9 8 7 6 5 4 3 2 1

Contents

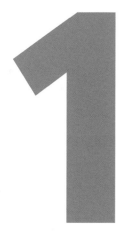

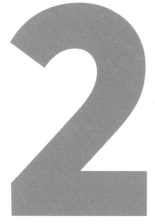

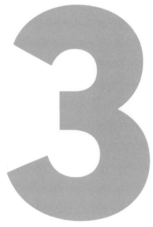

Your 90-Day Challenge

Rethinking Food & Diet

1

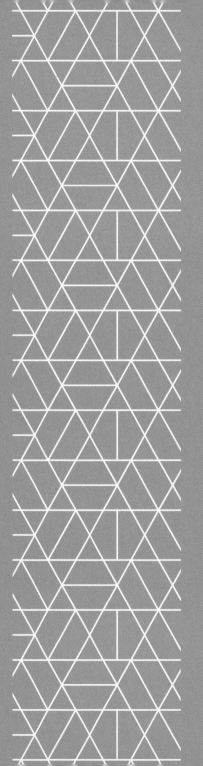

Your Best Self Starts Here

You are what you eat. Seriously. I know, it can be a hard concept to grasp, but when you consider that every ounce of your being—every cell, molecule, and structure—is miraculously constructed based on past food choices, it's both daunting and inspiring. Our day-to-day intake determines future outcomes—for better or for worse—and the beautiful thing about this process is that you get to decide what that looks like. Yes, you! Once you become fully aware that every bite and every sip taken in, and every drop of sweat poured out, creates the you that you're fully capable of becoming, then the wheels of change can begin to turn.

Don't feel overwhelmed or alone if your best self is lost at the moment, enveloped in poor food choices, drowning in drink, or way too familiar with time spent on the couch. It is still there, just waiting to be liberated from the depths and shepherded toward full potential. You have the power to take back control of your diet, food habits, and sweat sessions and pour your energy into becoming the person that you want to be. Start investing in yourself and explore what you are capable of when you reach for better choices.

Eating well can help us feel great and enjoy life more. So how is it that we keep getting this wrong? Perhaps we feel dazed by the vast availability and variety of food. Or we succumb to mixed messages surrounding food and nutrition. Given that every day presents us with food around every corner, on every counter, and at every meeting—and every social media feed depicts glorious plates of food and mixed messages of what to eat (or not) and when—we've earned the right to feel totally overwhelmed. So on the rare occasion when we get the quantity or timing or setting right, it's still easy to eat all the "wrong" foods. How we feel determines what we eat. It's no wonder that a majority of us no longer feel comfortable with our food choices or with our pants size.

We often set ourselves up for failure when we eat in response to emotion. Remember, nutrition itself is a science. If you can shift to viewing food as a way to find energy and nutrients and learn what comprises the best choices, then your best self can begin to take form, built on a platform of functional and powerful foods. This journal will equip you with essential information to help you build a strong nutritional foundation, day in and day out, rooted in deep-seated habits that play out as healthy choices. Change how you think about food and you will no longer be rocked by overeating, cravings, and emotions. Use this journal to put some distance between your feelings and how you fuel. Healthy eating can become a reality if you invest a little planning and intention.

I'm here as your nutrition coach. As a registered dietitian, I have helped countless individuals reach for better, and whether you've got a decent handle on nutrition or you're a complete disaster, I can help. No judging—I promise. I have seen it all, and I want to share what I've learned in a way that provokes thought and change in your life. Set aside 90 days for this journey. I will guide you to create new habits and make better food choices, and along the way, you will glean insights on why these choices matter. You'll need to commit to work: taking the time to track what you eat, keeping an open mind and experimenting to find an approach that works best for you, patiently putting it into practice, avoiding the common culprits, and getting up each time you fail. Take it one bite at a time, one week at a time, and the seemingly huge task of self-improvement will become more manageable.

Whether you're focused on getting to a healthy weight, fueling better athletic performance, cleaning up your diet, or simply hitting macronutrient goals, I promise you, you're in good hands.

I often hear, "I'll bet you have the perfect diet. You seem so regimented and perfect." If only that were true! Food intake isn't as simple as knowing *what* to eat . . . so many factors influence the when, where, and why. Even if my diet were pristine, imparting nutrition information is not as simple as modeling my perfect plate. Every plate will be different because it needs to suit *your* needs, *your* wants (within reason, of course), and *your* taste buds. What's on my plate shouldn't matter to you. I have to work every damn day to make better choices, just like you. To balance my intake with my output. To choose more color and fewer processed foods. While I love vegetables, I'm human too. When I get home after a stressful day, an adult beverage and salty food calls to me too. As do cake, cookies, and late-night eating. So I get you. Know that I fall off the wagon more than I'd like to admit. But no matter how many times that may happen, what's important is that we get back up, dust ourselves off, and try again.

Over the years, I've guided many people who were once clueless about which foods to put in their grocery cart, and even if they had a clue, they wouldn't know what to do with these foods when they got home. I'll give you a taste of basic nutrition, and explain the foods you need to fuel health and performance. Over the coming weeks and months, it will all meld together to give you the confidence you need to create change.

You are built on the <u>foods you choose</u>. Choose to build a <u>strong foundation</u>.

From there, it's time to set your personal goals. You might already have a nutrition or health goal in mind. Lose five pounds . . . and then some. Trade fat for muscle. Or maybe your intake and output don't seem to match up and you're desperate for some motivation to get to the gym more than once a week. Maybe you're a nutritional train wreck and need a complete overhaul. We will get down to the nitty-gritty to determine what drives your choices and what's holding you back, identify your specific nutritional pitfalls and personal obstacles, and evaluate your daily food choices.

Keep a Food Journal

Nutrition experts have long known that there's a simple tool anyone can use to improve their food choices, listen to their hunger cues, and ultimately improve their relationship with food. Food journals—or any method of logging your daily diet, whether online or on the back of a napkin—can be used to rein in portions, identify your emotional triggers, and help you reach your healthy weight. A recent study of 1,700 overweight or obese people conducted by the Kaiser Permanente Center for Health Research found that food journals are a helpful ally in the quest for weight loss: **Dieters who kept a food diary for six months lost twice as much weight as those who kept no food record.** Writing down what you eat makes you accountable for everything you eat and drink, including drive-by snacks, what's left of your kid's dinner, and pieces of chocolate. Food journals can also help reduce one of the biggest obstacles to meeting our goals: mindless and emotional eating. After all, if you have to measure out and log whatever food or drink you typically use to drown your sorrows, there's a good chance you'll get in touch with your emotions rather than cope with calories.

A food journal can also help you keep an eye on foods that you need to watch for optimal health—whether it's bad guys like sugar, good guys like fiber, calcium, and iron, or intolerances such as gluten or lactose. When you review what you ate in a day or a week, you can spot gaps in your intake, which could potentially deprive you of important nutrients. For example, if you get to the end of the day and see only one serving of vegetables (maybe just the lettuce on your sandwich), you'll realize that you're far from reaching your daily recommended intake! Find out if you're eating far more processed foods and fast foods than you'd like and whether these foods are replacing healthier, nutrient-dense choices. Keeping a food journal can also help you plan ahead for balanced meals and result in improved nutrition for everyone who eats at your table. And when you get discouraged, flipping back through your journal will allow you to see how far you've come.

Put in Some Sweat Equity

It's been said that you can't run from your problems, but I say you can. So if you're looking for an answer to your health, weight, or wellness questions, know that you're going to need to change more than just your diet. You're going to need to change your outfit too. Because the answers to whatever conundrum you're dealing with likely lie within the confines of Spandex, Dri-FIT, and any technical gear that accompanies a sweat session. That's right—look to exercise to resolve what's ailing you.

Habitual exercise has been clinically proven to have a positive impact on many conditions, from chronic and long-term to acute and temporary. It's critical in the fight against obesity, elevated blood lipids, and hypertension and results in a lower risk of cardiovascular disease, Alzheimer's disease, type 2 diabetes mellitus, eight types of cancer, and the list goes on. A most effective remedy, habitual exercise has the power to offer outcomes that often surpass those of prescription medications. Meanwhile, side effects are relatively benign, ranging from hurts-so-good muscle soreness to cramping your ability to binge-watch TV. Still, despite these familiar health benefits, physical *inactivity* remains a global pandemic—a disease striking every corner of the globe that has been called out as one of the four leading contributors to premature mortality. No longer are we falling prey to death by smoking; we're succumbing to death by sitting. I wonder, does the sedentary population realize the power of exercise? Aside from promoting better sleep quality and keeping triglycerides and blood glucose levels in check, sweat sessions fight off anxiety and depression and are uniquely able to provide a release—an escape from the overflowing inbox, the incessant requests of coworkers, the voice that tells you to drown your stress in sugary treats. For the short and sacred time we spend sweating, we're able to walk away from whatever may be hitting the fan and press pause on our vices.

For me, exercise is a constant companion to help me pilot a clearer course through everyday relationships, work, and conflict. It lends an ear and offers clarity when I'm problem-solving or working on an article. It's been my ally in the fight against poor food choices and faulty coping mechanisms. And those running endorphins have been solace for my soul, carrying me through the loss of loved ones, a heartbreaking stillbirth, and other dark corners of life.

But while movement is as simple as one foot in front of the other, the immersion that leads to routine sweat sessions is a complex process that is influenced by demographic, biological, cognitive, emotional, sociocultural, and environmental factors.

Each of us faces different barriers to making exercise a reality— schedule, family dynamics, budget, the recommended check-in with a doc before beginning a new program, or any list of potential obstacles that can prevent us from getting and staying active. Still, expert bodies like the American College of Sports Medicine (ACSM) remain entrenched in their recommendation that "a program of regular exercise that includes cardiorespiratory, resistance, flexibility, and neuro-motor exercise training beyond activities of daily living to improve and maintain physical fitness and health is essential for most adults." Getting started and keeping active isn't always as simple, but because it's essential to health and well-being, there are established set recommendations to guide our journey.

So, how much exercise is really necessary to reap the benefits? The answer to that question is *it depends*. If your goal is to move from a state of fairly sedentary to a place of habitual exerciser, then the recommendations that follow are something to reach for. You may not hit the total recommended weekly minutes for all types of exercise, falling short in some recommendations and meeting others. Or you might just be getting started, unfamiliar with all the different types of exercise and not yet accruing time across moderate, vigorous, strength, and flexibility. And that's okay. Your goal is ever forward—to get moving, develop a plan, and set out on a path so you can build toward meeting these recommendations.

If your goal is to stay relatively healthy and fight all-cause mortality, the guidelines provided by experts advising the United States Department of Health & Human Services and published in *Physical Activity Guidelines for Americans*, 2nd edition, are just what you need. Make sure you're hitting the recommendations listed on p. 11 and, over time, work for better. Take time to congratulate yourself for moving more and map out a course for progress. Stay motivated with some of these tips and never let those running shoes, walking shoes, or gym shoes accumulate dust.

If your goal is to go fast, get fitter, and strive for better performance, then it's time to work for it. Meet the recommendations and then aim for greater amounts of vigorous-intensity exercise, more dynamic workouts, and challenging sweat sessions (within reason, of course!).

Remember to cycle in various types of training blocks, like purposeful sessions focused on volume or intensity or even recovery. So if you've had months and years of logging the same mileage, at the same pace, and over the same terrain, then it's understandable that results would be, well, the same. When your goal is to seriously push your results, your training needs to take it up a notch, too.

Making Workouts Work
Find a Friend

Exercise is easier, more enjoyable, and more sustainable with someone by your side. One of my clients is a collegiate athlete turned mom and a corporate professional. It might seem that a former athlete would have no trouble making workouts happen, but she came to the realization that she needed external motivation and accountability to be consistent. Having a workout buddy and running partner means you have someone relying on you to be by their side and make them a better person too. It's easier to roll out of bed and show up for early morning runs, long rides, or a kettlebell session at the gym with a friend. After all, we all need someone to commiserate with!

Stop Feeling Selfish

Your health and personal goals often take a back seat to the needs of others. Quiet the voices that say you're neglecting something or someone simply because you took a well-deserved moment to focus on you. You are a better version of you in the hours post-workout. More positive and upbeat? Check. Feeling in-the-swing-of-things and able to tackle bigger tasks? You bet. An efficient and hardworking employee/spouse/parent? Check. Inspired to do more with each day? Yup. A better role model? Bingo. If you're run-down, stressed-out, or unhealthy, start by prioritizing self-care, and I promise you will be better able to care for others.

How intense is your sweat session?

Moderate

You feel the burn but can carry on a conversation.

×3–6 METs

Brisk walking

Recovery or light running

Leisurely cycling (<14 mph)

Easy swimming for fitness

Recreational sports with your kids

Carrying or moving heavy loads

Dancing

Intense indoor and outdoor housework (isn't it all intense?)

Vigorous

You are sweating and working too hard to have a conversation.

×6+ METs

Race walking

Running (speed work and tempo)

Cycling (18–20+ mph), hill climbing

Fast swimming (racing, speed work)

Competitive team sports (sprinting, start and stop)

High-intensity interval training

Barre classes, hot yoga

Strenuous strength sessions

Metabolic equivalents (METs) are commonly used to express the intensity of physical activities. This unit of measure is the ratio of your working metabolic rate relative to your resting metabolic rate. (See p. 69 for how to determine your RMR.)

One MET is defined as the energy cost of sitting quietly and is equal to a calorie burn of 1 calorie per kilogram of body weight per hour. It is estimated that compared with sitting quietly, caloric consumption is three to six times higher when being moderately active (3–6 METs) and more than six times higher when being vigorously active (>6 METs).

Just Do It Already

I've used just about every excuse out there to put off a run (which is ironic because I really love running). I eventually head out the door for an 18-mile turned 12-mile . . . no, make that a 6-mile run. Consequently, I run every race in an undertrained and underprepared state. Maybe you're a guilt-racked procrastinator too. Stop spinning your wheels and set a timer, make a to-do list, and get out the door. Use the sweat-session time to plan the rest of your day and you're sure to arrive home with a plan in place and a solid hit of confidence.

Start a Workout Habit

Research has shown that exercising at least four times a week for six weeks is the minimum investment needed to establish an exercise habit. When we work out, we rely on a combination of conscious intention (like planning to go and packing to go to the gym) and unconscious activities (like the habit of always going to the gym in the morning before work) operating in parallel to get us moving. Social cognitive theorists propose that it's our conscious intention that's the strongest predictor of whether or not we'll keep showing up; habit is possibly the strongest unconscious determinant of behavior. But the impact of planning and executing isn't immediate, so it's natural to fall off the workout wagon when you first begin. Instead of starting and stopping and starting and stopping, make it a goal to exercise X times per week and pledge to meet this goal for half of your *Sweat. Eat. Repeat.* journey. I promise you that consistent hard work will stick.

Make an Appointment

Feel yet another day slipping away without any sign of time for exercise? It's time to make an appointment. Just like you'd set aside time for an important project or meeting, block out some time for your workout. In a perfect world, you'd work out at the same time of the day and on

Rules of engagement for exercise

Even though hitting the recommended weekly exercise goals can lead to immediate benefits and regular activity has been associated with the prevention of at least 25 chronic diseases and health conditions, most people don't even come close. It's easy enough to lay out the recommendations and much harder to make it happen in real life. Even if you're not yet able to meet all of the targets outlined here, don't let it deter you. Benefits follow even the smallest amounts of exercise.

1
Move more and sit less. Some exercise is better than none, and benefits arise after as few as five minutes!

2
Commit to moderate-intensity cardio exercise for 150 to 300 minutes a week and accumulate this time over several days.

3
If vigorous activity is more your speed, accumulate 75 to 150 minutes of high-intensity cardio exercise a week. For best results, spread this activity throughout the week.

4
Find time for strength training. Two to three days each week, purposefully work each of the major muscle groups, including exercises designed to improve balance, agility, and coordination.

5
Don't forget to stretch. Assure joint range of movement by completing a series of flexibility exercises for each of the major muscle-tendon groups. Do each movement for a combined total of 60 seconds.

6
Personalize it. Every exercise program should be modified according to your habitual physical activity, physical function, health status, exercise responses, and, of course, personal goals.

the same days of the week. If you're able to be consistent, great. If your schedule needs to flex, that's fine too. The most important thing is to make time to become a better you.

Get Out of a Rut

Not seeing the performance gains you're looking for? It may be time to switch things up and add in bouts of high-intensity interval training (HIIT). At the baseline or beginning of a fitness journey, significant improvements in general fitness and overall endurance take place following moderate (for you fitness geeks out there, technically referred to as "submaximal") endurance training, *but* if you are highly trained and very fit, simply adding additional sessions (i.e., more volume) of moderate exercise does not appear to improve performance or fitness markers (like VO_2max or other physiological markers). Instead, researchers have found that for athletes who are already trained, improvements in endurance performance can be achieved only through HIIT. Nerd alert! These improvements are probably due to an increase in skeletal muscle buffering capacity rather than a change in oxidative or glycolytic enzyme activity.

Don't Undo the Workout

"If the fire is hot enough, anything will burn" is the slogan of athletes who prefer donuts and French fries to salad and grilled chicken. But it's the wrong approach. Exercise doesn't make us invincible, and the words *inflammation* and *cholesterol* exist whether you're just getting started or already on the podium. There's no escaping the fact that the foods you choose to power you through your day determine more than just your energy levels. Your choices impact health, wellness, weight, performance, and more. Think of it this way: If you want to drive a beater car, then the cheapest fuel will get you where you need to go. It's unlikely that you will enjoy the ride or make a great impression when you arrive, but you'll still make it from point A to point B. But why go through life piloting a car that starts and stalls when you could be experiencing a luxury ride? With premium fuel, every mile you cover will bring more enjoyment and enhanced performance, and you'll turn some heads too. So along with striving for better training and outcomes, make sure your food choices are supporting your fitness efforts. Don't fall victim to the common mistake of overeating your workout burn. And if you're filling up on crap, your health and performance will be crap. My friend, you are better than that.

An Eating Plan That Works. For You.

If you consider *diet* a four-letter word, you're not alone. Even uttering the word can induce emotional distress. While some diets serve little purpose other than to make you miserable while you attempt to shed pounds (e.g., a cabbage-soup diet or lemon-water detox), other diets give you a chance to try out a new lifestyle. Maybe that's why more than one-third of Americans in a recent weighted survey reported following one within the past year, which is up from 14 percent over the previous year. The majority of people following a diet are looking to restrict carbs and calories in one way or another. While diet popularity ebbs and flows, at this point in time, intermittent fasting is the most popular approach to dieting followed by paleo, low-carb, Whole30®, high-protein, and ketogenic or high-fat diet.

Let's take a fresh look at these diets—after all, your nutritional needs and goals might line up with a popular diet. In reality, whatever you eat from day to day makes up your personal diet. Many of us can benefit from one of these popular approaches or "prescriptive" diets because we just want someone to tell us what to eat already! Whether we are busy, confused, or stressed, a detailed diet provides some rules around food. Decision fatigue is a real thing and for good reason—we're inundated with food options 24/7. And while there is always willpower, we can only take so much before we break.

That's why today's lifestyle diets can work for some of us. On one side of the coin, they eliminate food groups or ingredients—and possibly nutrients if you're not careful—or restrict eating to specific times of the day. On the other side of the coin, they force you to carefully plan and consider every bite you consume. These prescriptions both take and give control. Certainly, they take away your ability to choose whatever you want to eat. But in return, they can give you feelings of accomplishment and empowerment, and in a roundabout way, they can lead to a lifestyle where you have more control over your health, your insatiable appetite, your waistline, or your day.

Which one to choose? That depends on you and what you're looking for. There is no "perfect diet" for everyone, and a pattern that works within the constraints of your current schedule and goals may not be the pattern that works for you in a year's time. And that's okay. While each of us may be searching for the one diet to rule them all, we are all different, and we all change over time. **The best diet for you is the one you can stick with long-term, the one that brings you positivity, the one that improves your health, and the one that helps you feel more comfortable around food.**

While some diets are designed to bring about holistic benefits, others are focused on weight loss. Still others result in combined health, wellness, and weight benefits. Choose a plan with the potential to help you improve what matters most to you. Some of these choices provide hard-and-fast rules, while others provide guardrails so you can fill up your plate as you see fit. Consider the pros and cons of each, and if you're still not sure which one could help you reach your goals, consider some of the fact-based info listed within these pages. And if, at the end of the day, you decide to chart your own course, that's fine too. One more thing: If you decide that one of these diets can help you reach your goals, be confident in your selection. After all, you're not alone in wishing that you didn't have so many damn decisions to make.

An Eating Plan That Works. For You.

Intermittent Fasting

For most people, even the idea of fasting evokes pangs of hunger and extreme thirst. Historically, people have fasted for religious reasons or in advance of a medical test. More recently, the concept of regular fasting for short periods of time, dubbed intermittent fasting, has become a popular tactic for achieving weight loss. Fans of intermittent fasting claim the practice leads to weight loss as well as mental clarity, an ability to focus on the task at hand without the distraction of eating, improved blood sugar control, and more.

➤ Here's How It Works

Intermittent fasting is not a diet per se but more of an eating schedule purported to have an effect on metabolism and accelerate fat loss and muscle growth. This plan has many variations, which we will take a look at, but it essentially requires you to eat within a certain window of time and fast for the remainder of the day. Both biology and human behavior demonstrate ways in which the circadian clock is involved in hormonal balance, including the appetite-regulating hormones leptin and ghrelin, which are subject to these day-night patterns. Studies have shown that consuming more energy earlier in the day aligns more closely with our circadian clock. We disrupt these rhythms with late-night snacking or bingeing after a stressful day at the office, which can lead to elevated blood sugar levels following a meal and even a greater risk of type 2 diabetes and obesity. **By promoting a drastically reduced "feeding window," intermittent fasting eliminates the opportunity to cram in needless energy right before bed.** Behaviorally, this approach can lead to weight loss for anyone who tends to mindlessly snack when bored, stressed, happy, and so forth. I'm not pointing fingers here! After all, we are all subjected to an overwhelming amount of social and emotional cues that drive us to eat until we are numb, so setting a schedule is helpful. In addition to effectively reducing calorie intake, intermittent

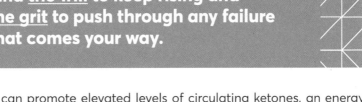

Find <u>the will</u> to keep rising and <u>the grit</u> to push through any failure that comes your way.

fasting can promote elevated levels of circulating ketones, an energy source for the brain and muscles when carbohydrate stores run low (read more about ketones in the section on ketogenic diet on p. 21). The benefits of ketones are varied, including the potential for enhanced cognition as well as reduced hunger and appetite.

➤➤ What Does the Science Say?

Time-restricted fasting: This variation of intermittent fasting limits food within specific time windows, such as 8:00 p.m. to 10:00 a.m. In this type of fasting, you spend the majority of the day in a fasted state. Popular methods include the 16:8 method, which would require you to consume your daily macro needs within an eight-hour window and fast for the rest. A more liberal ratio would be 12:12, and on the other extreme, some propose a ratio of 20:4, which is clearly not for the faint of heart.

Research suggests that this method can lead to reductions in fasting glucose and improvements in LDL and HDL cholesterols. Understandably, self-reported hunger was higher in the morning for those consuming a single meal per day, and subjects did not report becoming accustomed to this hunger over the course of the study.

Alternate-day fasting: This approach entails alternating between fasting and feasting every other day. On a "fast day," you can consume energy-free fluids, and on a "feast day," you can eat whatever you want.

Research published in the *Journal of the American Medical Association* comparing people who participated in alternate-day fasting to those on a standard, reduced-calorie diet found that there was no difference in weight loss or weight maintenance between the two groups over the course of one year. Begging the question, is compliance to frequent full-day fasts reasonable and, even more important, exactly how far off the rails did subjects go on feast days?

All in all, this style of IF may lead to modest weight loss with possible improvement in metabolic parameters, but hunger on fast days is intense and does not always wane over time.

Modified fasting: Sometimes referred to as 5:2 intermittent fasting, this approach to intermittent fasting involves eating a typical diet five days a week and then limiting your food intake to 20 to 25 percent of your caloric needs on two nonconsecutive days. In other words, if you follow an 1,800-calorie diet, you would eat 1,800 calories five days a week and about 450 calories or less on restricted days.

Research suggests that this method results in weight loss, with modest and mixed effects on blood sugar control, blood lipid levels, and inflammatory markers. However, a review and a randomized clinical trial concluded that there is little evidence to suggest that this method produces superior weight loss or metabolic changes in comparison to standard energy restriction regimens.

➤➤ Should You Try It?

If you struggle because food controls every minute of your day and you need a hard break, then yes, give IF a try. Or if you are looking for hard-and-fast rules around when to eat, IF could be for you. Or if you're looking to promote higher levels of circulating ketones and want to tap into that alternate fuel source, IF could open doors. But if you've tried (intentionally or accidentally) skipping meals only to find that you overeat when food is once again available, a steadier intake of fuel may be a better choice for you. Rob Klingensmith, an endurance athlete and owner of the Lens Agency, found that a variation of IF with hard-and-fast rules of what to eat the rest of the day works best for him. His plan? No food after 8:00 p.m. and nothing but coffee until 10:00 a.m., with a set plan in place for when it's time to eat. To meet his goal of improved body composition, he follows a macronutrient-focused 40/30/30 (carbs/protein/fat) plan with some indulgences on the weekends. "I found a way of eating that lets me enjoy some of my favorite foods, fuels my performance, yet keeps me on track—the best of both worlds."

For cardio junkies or anyone actively training for an event or cranking through intense workouts on a regular basis, IF is probably not the best choice. Research shows that intense forms of fasting are likely detrimental to aerobic athletic gains; calories consumed in the hours before a workout are essential for optimal performance, recovery, and muscle gain.

➤➤ Know Before You Go

Intermittent fasting is heavily promoted to athletes and fitness enthusiasts as a way to achieve and maintain a very lean, strong physique. Many of the benefits—such as improved body composition and mental focus—remain primarily anecdotal, and there's no robust science to support these claims. In other words, there's no magic at work here. The reason IF may work has more to do with calorie restriction than a metabolic makeover. Intermittent fasting with caloric restriction often yields equivalent benefits as traditional low-calorie diets in regard to changes in fat mass, improving insulin sensitivity, and improving blood lipid profiles. Elevated levels of circulating ketones may provide an alternate source of energy and thus have the added benefit of alleviating discomfort due to low energy.

If you're looking for quick results and adaptation, IF may not be for you as it can take a few days (or longer) to adjust to this way of fueling.

This period of adaptation can be very uncomfortable as restricted eating has been anecdotally associated with extreme hunger, irritability, loss of strength, loss of libido, and other negative side effects. But once you get used to IF, your hunger levels may decrease, and your mood could become more positive compared to before the fasting program started. But that's *if* you get used to it. Some studies have found a higher dropout rate among intermittent fasters, suggesting it might not be a sustainable approach.

Also, IF is not a food free-for-all. All the approaches outlined above emphasize the importance of the nutritional quality of the meals that are consumed. Nutrients such as protein, fat, fiber, vitamins, and minerals are essential for good health, and since nutrients are not consumed while fasting, they are especially important when breaking the fast. In addition, drinking a lot of water is encouraged both to stay hydrated and to alleviate hunger.

Dr. Chris Mohr, a nutrition expert and the co-owner of Mohr Results, a well-being consulting company, suggests the following for successful IF: Keep your foray into IF short so you don't slow your metabolism, remember that your feeding window is not an opportunity for a feeding frenzy, focus on protein in order to maintain your muscle while losing weight and also to stay satisfied, and, finally, since your quantity of food is limited, make sure you're focusing on quality. If you regularly find yourself wishing for food rather than focusing on the task at hand or avoiding social activities, look for a different approach to reach your goals.

HOW TO MAKE INTERMITTENT FASTING WORK FOR YOU

Don't get stuck searching for the perfect IF plan. Research suggests that all variations offer the benefit of extreme caloric control that will lead you to reconceptualize hunger. Instead of allowing hunger to trigger panic, think about it as a chance to show off your willpower as you stick to your plan.

Set a workout-fasting schedule so you can enjoy a complete post-workout meal and recover more effectively.

To get the most out of your workout, add in some caffeine and supplemental branched-chain amino acids (BCAAs) beforehand. The caffeine lowers your rate of perceived exertion so the workout won't feel as strenuous, while the BCAAs in your bloodstream can help preserve muscle glycogen and protein stores during the workout, leading to lower risk of bonking, less soreness, and better recovery.

Don't fill up on crap calories. Overdo it on pizza, fried foods, and donuts on nonfasting days (or hours) and you surpass your calorie needs and miss out on the nutrients your body needs to be at its best. Have a plan and work it.

Don't go overboard. If you become overzealous and develop a poor relationship with food, it's time to step away from IF (and diet plans in general) and seek the advice of a nutrition expert.

The Ketogenic Diet

If an exponential increase in Google search rankings, a multitude of innovations on the market, and the rise in prices of related in-demand, high-fat foods are an indication of the diet du jour, then keto is certainly having its day in the sun.

The ketogenic diet is not a new diet; it's a high-fat, adequate-protein, very low-carb lifestyle that's been used for decades to treat epileptic seizures as well as other chronic conditions, such as metabolic syndrome. The premise is this: By severely restricting carbohydrates, the body is forced to either find an alternate source of fuel or perish. Survival mode and evolution kicks in, and instead of being a carb-burning machine, relying on blood sugar for fuel and the pancreas and insulin to utilize said fuel, the body transitions to burning fat stores and dietary fat as the liver creates a source of fuel known as ketones. When this happens, the body enters a metabolic state known as ketosis, in which the body's energy supply comes from ketone bodies in the blood. This is in direct contrast to the native state of glycolysis, in which blood glucose provides most of the energy.

➤➤ Here's How It Works

On your plate, keto looks like high-fat butter-coffee and a cheesy omelet topped with avocado and bacon for breakfast, a lettuce-wrapped burger for lunch, and a ribeye steak topped with sautéed mushrooms and creamed spinach for dinner. In other words, hold the grains, bread, fruit, and craft beer.

Ketogenic diets work for a multitude of reasons: There is both a metabolic shift and a reduction in overall calorie intake at play. Given the severe carb restriction, ketogenic diets do not allow for intake of empty-calorie, high-sugar treats, nor do they allow for an overwhelming choice of foods. Many dieters stick to their plan and rarely surpass calorie goals because their options are limited. What's the point of butter without popcorn or guac without tortilla chips? In addition, the elimination of carbs ultimately reduces blood sugar fluctuations, decreases appetite, and significantly reduces hunger signals.

Physiologically, the diet is effective because it disrupts the usual state of glycolysis, which is when circulating insulin promotes storage of body fat and blocks the release of fatty acids from adipose tissue. Instead, in a ketogenic state, fat reserves are readily released and consumed as ketone production occurs. These ketone bodies can then be used by the brain and muscle tissue as a fuel source to replace some of the needs originally supplied by glucose. This is why ketosis is sometimes referred to as the body's "fat-burning" mode.

⇥ What Does the Science Say?

The exact definition of a ketogenic diet in terms of carbohydrate pre-scription may vary slightly, but published studies and texts agree that the diet should be designed around the following principles:

An extremely limited carbohydrate intake: Supplying less than 20 to 50 grams of carbohydrates per day. That's less than 5 to 10 percent of your total daily calorie intake.

Adequate protein to support lean body needs: Approximately 0.5 to 0.7 grams of protein per pound of lean mass (i.e., you don't feed the extra weight you hope to shed!). This should total about 20 percent of your total daily calories.

High in fat: Supplying about 75 percent of daily calories. Overall, your daily intake should supply at least two times as much fat compared to every *combined* gram of protein and carbs. For example, if you consume 10 grams of fat, you would eat no more than 5 grams of a mix of protein and carbs and choose protein first since it's more ketogenic than carbs.

While many endurance athletes are practically baptized on bagels and drowning in gels and energy bars, six-time world Ironman® cham-pion Dave Scott has turned to the ketogenic diet as a way to fuel his health and performance. A major shift from his days of being spon-sored by sports drinks and bananas, Scott now believes in, personally consumes, and recommends a low-carb, high-fat approach to eat-ing. He has observed that this satiating, steady-energy diet has led to improvements in performance, health parameters, and even body composition. His appetite is reduced as a result of getting his body into a state of ketosis.

Science supports Scott's opinion: Ketosis regulates two key hormones, ghrelin and leptin, which signal hunger or fullness. When it comes to weight loss and improvements in body composition, multiple research studies have found keto to be effective. One study established that a low-calorie ketogenic diet results in both fast and longer-term weight loss. This study compared effects of a low-calorie ketogenic diet (LCKD) versus a standard low-calorie diet (LCD). The LCKD resulted in significant effects on body weight at 6, 12, and 24 months. At 24 months, the diet brought even greater reductions in body weight, waist circumference, and body-fat mass. In those who completed the program, there were significant effects on weight loss at 2 weeks, 2 months, 4 months, 6 months, 1 year, 1.5 years, and 2 years.

And as for overall health? A study of 46 men compared the effects of two different diets where energy intake and output offset each other: a very high-fat, low-carb diet (73% fat / 17% protein / 10% carbohydrates) versus a low-fat, high-carb diet (30% fat / 17% protein / 53% carbohydrates). Both caloric-restriction diets led to improvements in weight (loss of 12 kg versus 11 kg, respectively), but the keto diet showed more significant total health (circulating metabolic markers) improvements after just 8 weeks, as compared to 12 weeks for other diets. And weight loss on this plan is typically quick; in this study, dieters lost 4.8 kg (10.5 lb.) during the first four weeks. The plan has support from experts like Fredrick J. Stare, professor of nutrition and epidemiology at the renowned Harvard T.H. Chan School of Public Health: "The low-fat diet backfired. American's obesity epidemic skyrocketed even while our fat intake went down."

However, not all of the research on the ketogenic diet is positive and not all clinicians advocate for this restrictive approach to eating. While dieters enjoy keto because it allows intakes of some of their favorite foods that they once believed to be forbidden, clinicians criticize the diet for severely restricting or eliminating whole grains, fruit, and other choices, and they question it as a long-term approach to health and wellness. As a registered dietitian, I have seen the positive effects this diet can bring about for weight loss, for quieting sugar cravings and appetite, and for those struggling with chronic diseases. But I've also counseled plenty of clients through side effects like dehydration, electrolyte losses, fatigue, micronutrient deficiencies, negative impact on blood lipid levels, and general difficulty with making it work.

If you want to try keto, know that over the short term, it's likely a harmless approach to quick weight loss. The clinical trials investigating its long-term safety in general populations are limited at this time, but it appears safe past 36 months. Any research looking beyond three years is concentrated on pediatric, epileptic populations and should not be translated to generally healthy adults. While the ketogenic diet is great for quick weight loss, you'll want to think twice before you land on it as the be-all, end-all diet for life. While some studies suggest that adherence to a keto diet for up to 36 months far outpaces the acceptance of a low-fat diet, other studies have found that after the first few months of weight loss (three to six months), dieters begin to plateau, and the benefits of keto were similar to those of a low-carb or a 40/30/30 plan over a year's time.

➤ Should You Try It?

Are you looking for weight loss, less hunger and reduced appetite, and a steady level of energy? Are you willing to put in a few weeks of totally overhauling your diet before adapting to this way of fueling? If you're looking to lower your sugar intake, want to track your macros, and are willing to say no to your usual way of eating and fueling, then keto could be for you. People who benefit from keto often have significant weight to lose, but advocates of the diet also include individuals looking for better cognition and focus and those looking to improve metabolic markers and levels of inflammation.

An Eating Plan That Works. For You.

The benefits of keto for serious athletes have yet to be fully examined, and current research suggests that keto does not accelerate performance nor is it the right approach for athletes in high-intensity sports. So if you're looking to PR at your next 10K or if you're committed to a regimen of HIIT workouts, you might want to rely on good old glucose, which burns easily and without a high oxygen cost, rather than rely on ketones. That being said, many athletes who have transitioned to a ketogenic diet during the off-season and become keto-adapted, consistently relying on ketones for fuel, report performance improvements and finally getting to the elusive race-weight number.

➤➤ Know Before You Go

Keto is not for everyone, including those with a genetic risk for cardiovascular disease, certain metabolic conditions, and those who find that a high intake of saturated fat drives up their lipid levels. With so many viable choices out there, don't get frustrated if this is not the diet for you.

For individuals beginning the regimen, it often takes three to five weeks to transition. So don't wake up on Monday with a plan to start keto when you've got an important race on Friday. And don't give up on keto if you've only given it a few days to take hold. Many people following keto respond well to the food choices and guardrails put in place to achieve ketosis, yet others find keto to be too restrictive and eliminating of favorite foods. If you simply can't survive without fruit or pasta or you're not a fan of avocado, olive oil, bacon, coconut oil, MCT oil, and heavy cream, then you may want to think twice before diving in.

➤ HOW TO MAKE KETO WORK FOR YOU

The more strictly you follow this diet, the better. Because it takes days to adapt and burn off the glycogen you have on board, cheat days effectively restart the keto clock, and can also promote inflammation.

Sweat. Eat. Repeat.

Set aside a month to strictly follow the keto diet before you consider cyclical approaches or the slightest cheat day, says Robert Santos-Prowse, clinical registered dietitian and author of *The Ketogenic Mediterranean Diet* and *The Cyclical Ketogenic Diet*. After that, you can allow yourself "carb breaks"—like integrating some rice or fruit. Fall off the wagon entirely and it will take you a few days to restore ketosis. However, a few breaks here and there can help you to follow this lifestyle long-term.

Higher-fat and lower-carb intakes lead to better results. Macronutrient ratios closer to 5 percent of calories from carbs, 20 percent from protein, and 75 percent from fat will lead to higher levels of ketones, and the majority of the weight that is lost stems from fat mass rather than a loss of both fat and lean tissue.

Don't overdo the protein. Excess protein can undergo gluconeogenesis, a process where amino acids are converted to a source of blood glucose, which the body can then rely upon for fuel. To rely on ketones instead, you'll need to establish a protein intake that's adequate but not excessive.

Hydrate, hydrate, hydrate! The initial weight loss on this diet is due to diuresis or fluid loss. Dr. Carolyn Dean, a medical advisory board member of the Nutritional Magnesium Association, warns followers to hydrate and replace electrolytes or else suffer through dehydration and the effects that accompany it: headaches, fatigue, and feeling like you've got the keto flu. Dr. Dean recommends drinking half your body weight (in pounds) in ounces of water. Add ¼ teaspoon of sea salt or mineral-rich Himalayan salt to every quart of drinking water along with a teaspoon of magnesium citrate powder.

Plan ahead. You're probably not accustomed to filling up on fat, so you'll need to plan ahead to have the right foods available when hunger hits.

An Eating Plan That Works. For You.

Low-Carb Diets

If you've ever tried to follow a low-carb or a no-carb diet, you know that carbs are omnipresent. Seriously. They're seemingly in every food, in every sip and in every bite. Our bodies are designed to run quite efficiently and effectively on carbs, so the fact that this macronutrient is readily available is great for survival . . . or *was* great for survival. In today's world, carbs are both overabundant and overprocessed, contributing to an epidemic of excessive calories and an ever-expanding plate.

➤ Here's How It Works

Which came first? High-carb diets or expanding waistlines? With more than two-thirds of American adults being overweight or obese and with the average diet supplying approximately 50 percent of calories from carbohydrates, both consumers and experts are on the hunt for the answer to this question. The 1990s brought an emphasis on low-fat diets, which tipped the scales in favor of carbs, hooking people on processed foods riddled with sugar and meals overflowing with starchy filler. Now more than one-third of consumers across Europe and North America believe they should eat less bread, pasta, potatoes, and rice in the interest of weight and wellness. The emerging scientific view that carbohydrate intake is implicated in cardiovascular disease (via inflammation) as well as the suite of signs and symptoms indicative of metabolic syndrome is only fueling the outrage against glucose.

To understand the definition of "low-carb" you must first understand the intention behind the Acceptable Macronutrient Distribution Range (AMDR). Established by the National Academy of Medicine, the AMDR provides guidance around intake of the commonly tracked macros. These levels are based on decades of research (although some experts say these levels need some tweaking based on more current evidence) and suggest a range of macronutrient intake with the potential to reduce risk of chronic disease while still allowing for adequate intake of essential nutrients. The AMDR for carbohydrates is set at 45 to 65 percent of daily calories, so technically any diet that provides less than 45 percent of calories from carbs is characterized as low-carb. However, **many researchers and low-carb advocates suggest an intake much lower than 45 percent of daily calories is best.**

When it comes to the ever-popular low-carb approach, you can pick your poison. Each approach varies slightly from the next, with the diet founder putting their own spin on it. Some, like the Atkins diet and the Zone Diet or 40/30/30, have been around for decades, are well researched, and can lead to great outcomes. Others are less prescriptive, not clinically researched, and their outcomes are mostly anecdotal in nature.

➤➤ What Does the Science Say?

The war over the impact of low-carb diets on health and waistlines has been waged for decades. Some experts (disclaimer: not this expert) side with the recent *Lancet* report that low-carb diets lead to poor outcomes and an increase in mortality. This epidemiological study followed close to 15,500 people for three decades, checked in on them a few times, and asked subjects twice to articulate what they had eaten over the past year. Food-frequency questionnaires like the one used in this study are always tricky; most individuals can barely remember what they had for lunch let alone what they enjoyed for lunch five months ago! And favorite foods reported a decade ago are not necessarily reflective of foods consumed at points in between check-ins. In addition to limitations in reporting intake, the reported risks incurred by the individuals who consumed fewer carbs (less than 40 percent of calories from carbs) could have been related to other lifestyle choices; these individuals were more likely to smoke, exercise less, consume less fiber, and have a higher BMI. Not that the lower carbohydrate intake *caused* these factors—these are simply associations. Still, this large longitudinal trial is worth considering before you dive into a long-term, low-carb lifestyle. And there are some important takeaways: Diets that included higher intakes of plant-based protein and fat and less animal-based protein and fat often led to better outcomes. And while some experts disagree with the purported risks of going low-carb, we can all agree that consuming more plants and less animals can lead to better overall health outcomes.

So are your friends right when they tell you low-carb diets lead to skinny jeans and weight loss without hunger? Perhaps. A recent study published in the *BMJ* found that people who followed a low-carb diet burned more calories than those who consumed a high-carb diet. The study assigned overweight or obese individuals who had previously lost weight to one of three weight-maintenance diets: a high-carb diet (60 percent of calories from carbs), a moderate-carb diet (40 percent of calories from carbs), or a low-carb diet (20 percent of calories from carbs). After 20 weeks, individuals on the low-carb diet had burned 209 to 278 more calories a day than those on the high-carb diet. This translates to a metabolic shift of 50 to 70 calories a day for every 10 percent decrease in carbohydrate intake. Still another study compared the effects of a low-carb diet (less than 40 grams of carbs per day and a macro split of 34% carbs / 24% protein / 41% fat) to a low-fat diet (less than 30 percent of energy from fat with a macro split of 54% carbs / 19% protein / 29% fat) in terms of both weight loss and risk of cardiovascular disease. The dieters ate approximately the same amount of calories each day over one year's time. The low-carb group ended up losing almost three times as much weight as the low-fat group and experienced more significant improvements in body composition and other risk factors.

➤ Should You Try It?

If you're looking to manage appetite and reduce cardiovascular-risk markers, triglycerides, and circulating levels of insulin (a fat-depositing hormone) and are seeking improvements in fasting blood sugar levels and your overall body composition while also reducing the number on the scale—but want an approach that includes more variety than a ketogenic diet—a low-carb diet could be a good solution for you. However, while the effects of a low-carb diet are compelling, many of these benefits can arise from other ways of eating as well. And low-carb diets are not typically recommended for cardio junkies or for athletes in heavy training in pursuit of a new PR. These plans result in a reduction in glycogen stores (i.e., muscle fuel), so if your goal is to go fast and long, a low-carb diet isn't likely to get you there.

➤➤ Know Before You Go

Regardless of the percentage of calories from carbs or the limit of grams per day, when you follow a low-carb diet, you'll be restricting carbs while being more liberal with your intake of protein and fat. It's difficult to say whether it's the low-carbohydrate content of the diet or the high-protein content of the diet that drives the benefits. Research has looked at various levels of protein and carbohydrate combinations, and the effects of an increase in protein are not to be overlooked, as you'll see when we take a closer look at high-protein diets. All in all, if you're trying to lose weight or get lean and mean, the potential benefits of a well-designed low-carbohydrate diet are clear. But for overall health and well-being, it's important to note that many food groups are restricted or eliminated when you go low-carb. Watch for possible nutrient deficiencies of vitamins A, C, and E, as well as thiamine, B6, folate, calcium, magnesium, iron, potassium, and fiber. You can thwart these with creative meal planning as well as supplementation. In addition, due to diuresis and low fiber intake, you might find yourself suffering from headaches and constipation—common complaints that can be addressed with balanced choices, intake of electrolytes, and more fluids.

⇨ HOW TO MAKE A LOW-CARB DIET WORK FOR YOU

Swap starches for veggies as "better carbs." Try zucchini spirals, riced cauliflower, or lentil-based pastas.

Watch your overall calorie intake if you want to lose weight. Many foods that are rich in protein and fat can be rich in calories as well. If going back for seconds, grab veggies first and then protein.

Red-light, green-light foods. Try eliminating a problem food, such as bread or pasta, but allow sweet potatoes, quinoa, or lentils instead.

Ask yourself, "need" or "want"? Do you need that cookie, or do you want the cookie? You know the answer.

High-carb foods are cheap and plentiful, so plan ahead in order to have higher-protein and higher-fat foods ready when hunger calls.

High-Protein Diets

Are you going low-carb or high-protein (and is there a difference)? High-protein diets are typically followed by those who are looking to put on mass, prevent muscle loss, or gain strength. Other high-protein eaters are looking to get lean and replace fat mass with muscle, but not necessarily gain or lose weight. A high-protein diet is technically an intake above the recommended daily allowance (RDA), but at 0.8 grams per kilogram of body weight (~0.4 g/lb.), the RDA is so low that most all active individuals should aim to surpass it. Instead, many experts direct their clients to follow the AMDR, which specifies 10 to 35 percent of calories as coming from protein; an intake surpassing 35 percent constitutes a high-protein diet.

Low-carb vs. keto

Low-carb diets and keto diets are not the same thing, but it's entirely possible for them to arrive at similar end points. Chris Mohr, a nutrition expert, notes that virtually nothing has been debated more in the nutrition world than carbohydrates versus fats. And it seems that everyone is wondering which is better for weight loss and health. But Dr. Mohr says that it needn't be an issue of either/or: Instead of focusing on which one is better, we should ask, what are the similarities between the two approaches that can work for everybody? We can all agree that vegetables are important to a healthy diet and we should all consume an abundance of those. High-fiber berries and other low-glycemic fruits are also good choices, regardless of your eating plan. Whether you go keto or low-carb, focus less on ribeye, beef, and bacon and more on the opportunity to consume more salmon, berries, and avocados. Think about the long-term viability, overall variety, and adherence to the diet you choose because an option that works for your lifestyle is far more likely to work for you.

➤➤ Here's How It Works

Protein's role in weight maintenance stems from its potential to increase satiety and thermogenesis (which is an uptick in the metabolic cost of digestion) while also preserving metabolically active muscle tissue. In other words, any weight lost is more likely to be fat and not muscle. A higher intake of protein is also essential when cutting calories since the body will use protein for energy to create glycogen and to fulfill the host of other functions protein does throughout the day. This higher intake of protein also helps fend off hunger and appetite, which helps with adherence to the plan!

An Eating Plan That Works. For You.

Paleo, carnivore, and other all-meat-all-the-time diets fit this plan. Yes, these are also low-carb diets, so you can see the overlap here. The paleo diet includes foods that can be hunted, gathered, or fished in the great outdoors as opposed to hunted or gathered off the shelves at your local grocer! Really, this approach is more a lifestyle than a diet, rooted in the theory that our bodies are genetically programmed to eat like our caveman ancestors and that our genome has not yet adapted to many of the foods on the grocer's shelves; intake of modern, processed foods has resulted in inflammation and other chronic diseases. If you adopt this approach, you aren't limited to hunting for your supper, although the additional exercise could help you meet health goals faster! Today's paleo diet has been updated to include high intake of fresh vegetables and fruits; fresh items in the butcher's case (think grass-fed beef, wild-caught fish, free-range poultry and eggs); a moderate intake of nuts, berries, and honey; low intake of grains; and no dairy, legumes, alcohol, or refined carbohydrates. All in all, paleo is high in protein, low in carbs (since foods like starchy vegetables, grains, and sugar are eliminated), and relatively high in fiber.

The carnivore diet is a high-protein (low-carb) plan that could also be dubbed "the anti-vegan diet." This plan calls for calories from any cut of meat you can get your claws on. Higher-fat cuts of red meat, fish, eggs, organ meats, as well as some dairy and condiments are permissible. No fruits, vegetables, grains, or supplements are allowed, and proponents of the diet say that this very minimalistic approach to eating leads to a reduction in inflammation and an increase in overall health and longevity. Critics point out that with no produce or starches in your cart, this plan can cost a pretty penny, lead to nutritional deficiencies if followed long-term, and seriously disrupt your gut microbiome—starving both the good and the bad bacteria, while also wreaking havoc on your digestive regularity.

➤➤ What Does the Science Say?

While randomized clinical trials studying the effects of the paleo and the carnivore diets are limited or nonexistent, the impact of protein on weight loss has been studied ad nauseum. Anyone who's dieted knows that feeling hungry and restricted all the time does not lead to success (or happiness!). Enter protein with its proven ability to promote satiety and increase thermogenesis. **The metabolic increase of a higher-protein diet is related to the fact that the calorie cost to digest protein is generally greater than that of carbohydrates and fat,** which is yet another reason why high-protein diets can promote weight loss.

Generally, any body weight lost leads to a reduction in metabolism, since smaller mass requires less energy to maintain. Therefore, once you lose weight, you have to decrease your intake (or else you'll gain it all back). Because of its role in satiety and calorie burn, protein has been studied for its potential to moderate this reduction in energy expenditure. After a four-week weight-loss program, subjects participated in a three-month follow-up for weight maintenance, with half the group receiving an additional 48.2 grams of protein per day (an approximate 20 percent increase, with 18 percent instead of 15 percent of calories from protein). Participants with a modest bump in protein intake showed a 50 percent reduced regain of body weight lost and also reported feeling more full. And the weight that was regained in the protein group was predominantly lean mass, not fat mass, resulting in an overall lower percentage of body fat. This data suggests that even moderate increases in protein intake can help keep the weight off after a short-term weight-loss program.

➤➤ Should You Try It?

If you're looking to feel satiated longer while cutting calories or if you want to build, get lean, and recover from taxing HIIT and CrossFit®

workouts, then a high-protein diet can help. Just be sure to design your plate to include a mix of plant proteins and fats rather than rely solely on animal protein. Habitually high intakes of animal fats and proteins are linked to an increased risk of heart disease, excessive protein can tax kidney function, and these foods often lack some of the micronutrients and all of the fiber that's found in plants. In other words, skip the carnivore diet. For better digestive health and in the interest of losing a few inches, a varied diet that's high in protein and low in processed foods can be a good choice.

➤➤ Know Before You Go

If you want to avoid the muscle breakdown and loss that can accompany heavy activity or aging, or you want to avoid the all-too-familiar hunger that accompanies calorie restriction, aim to take in 30 percent or more of total calories from varied protein sources. Choose protein from whole food sources, such as lean meats, fish, poultry, and dairy as well as plant-based legumes and ancient grains, which increase your protein intake as well as overall nutrient and fiber intake.

➡ HOW TO MAKE A HIGH-PROTEIN DIET WORK FOR YOU

Skip starches and fill your plate with filling fiber-rich veggies and lean protein sources.

Include a source of protein every time you eat. Choose snacks with at least 15 grams of protein and meals with at least 30 grams, depending on your overall goals and calorie needs.

Vary your intake to assure you're getting a variety of amino acids as well as a variety of micronutrients.

Say it with me: "Protein powder is my friend." Protein powders draw from a variety of sources, and they taste good. Select one from a reputable brand that has 20 to 30 grams of protein per serving and less than 5 grams of carbs and fat.

High-carb and high-fat foods are the mainstay of drive-thru and restaurant menus, so you'll need to commit to planning and meal prep.

Detox Diets

The popularity of detox diets tends to follow the seasons; New Year's resolutions and swimsuit season are peak times for these approaches, which promise weight loss, total body wellness, or some other magic as a result of the removal of a buildup of toxins. There are many approaches to detox, ranging from 3-day juice fasts to 30-day detoxes, during which time dieters are instructed to eliminate certain food groups or to drink "cleansing" beverages daily. Nutrition expert Jenna Bell, PhD, RD, advises to be wary of any plan that promises fast, nearly overnight results and cuts out most every food group. "If your goal is long-term and sustainable weight loss, think before you leap because detoxes are unlikely to help you lose weight for good, yet are very likely to leave you feeling run-down as a result of missing nutrients. And at the end of the day, once you stop the detox, the weight is likely to return."

➤➤ Here's How It Works

Some of the intolerances or toxins linked with certain foods can get unruly when left unchecked—the culprits can be gluten, caffeine, pesticides, or alcohol, to name a few. Foods that are considered hard to digest and absorb, like meat, cheese, and processed foods, are often on the "do not eat" list and, in theory, as a result of avoiding these food items, the body uses less energy to digest food and fight off toxins. **By eliminating certain food groups, these diets target toxins associated with the eliminated foods, while also giving the digestive system a break.** Instead of using energy to digest and absorb, the body can redirect energy to healing and recovery.

➤➤ What Does the Science Say?

As you might have gathered, detox diets are better supported by behavioral science than data-driven research. I credit detox diets less for their ability to "detox" the body (since that's what your liver and kidneys are for) and more for their ability to provide a hard stop to any poor habits you just can't seem to break. Think of it this way: A three-day juice cleanse will force you to stop eating junk food because you're only "allowed" fluids.

Today's detox diets typically involve extreme restriction, the removal of certain food groups, or even daily consumption of "cleansing" beverages. The popular Whole30 diet is, in my mind, a detox diet. Whole30 focuses on eliminating specific food groups for one month— grains (which includes any starch, bran, or wheat germ you can think of), dairy, sugar (including honey, agave, maple syrup, and all non-nutritive sweeteners), alcohol, and all processed foods. Regular weigh-ins are discouraged (even though research suggests otherwise to stay focused on weight-related goals). Over time, foods are reintroduced slowly with the goal of identifying trigger foods and intolerances. Many followers of Whole30 anecdotally tout its ability to provide a break from food addictions and bring about a full-body "cleanse" because individuals often emerge from this restrictive plan with a better relationship with food and the ability to eat more intuitively—which I can definitely get behind! However, it's important to note that this uber-popular diet is based on theory and hearsay. For starters, it lacks the research to prove its claims because most people don't follow it long enough to effectively reduce inflammation. Furthermore, most nutrition experts (myself included) view Whole30 as restrictive, hard to follow, and deficient in fiber and many micronutrients.

➤➤ Should You Try It?

Detox diets can give you a break from bad habits or force you to ignore cravings. If you stick with the plan laid out before you, a short detox might help you build willpower and confidence. Just be careful you don't turn a three-day plan into a chronic practice of long-term restriction. Detox diets tend to severely limit calories, leaving you feeling weak, tired, and crappy. An occasional dip into detox probably won't hurt you, but these plans are not sustainable or healthy in the long run.

It's been my experience that active individuals with serious goals are better off avoiding detox plans. They may help you fit into skinnier jeans by the weekend, but they totally miss the bigger picture of helping you choose better. Better choices over time are what leads to health, wellness, and confidence. These plans don't equip you with real skill; they simply see how long you can hold on before you're forced to throw in the towel. Once you finish the 30-day detox and return to variation in your diet, you might find yourself with fewer cravings and "addictions," but the weight you worked so hard to lose is certain to return because most of the changes you made weren't sustainable. Detox diets epitomize research published in a report in *American Psychologist*, which says that while dieters can lose 5 to 10 percent of their body weight in the first few months of a diet, more than 60 percent will regain the weight they lose, and then some, within four or five years of ending the diet.

➤➤ Know Before You Go

Other than the fact that weight loss is temporary and restricting your intake is difficult, there are some real health concerns to be aware of before starting a detox diet. Short-term consequences can range

An Eating Plan That Works. For You.

from temporary feelings of lethargy and malaise to lingering physical harm from drug-nutrient interactions or potentially toxic components in cleansing products—in other words, skip commercially available detox products. People have been led astray hoping to thwart or cure chronic diseases, such as type 2 diabetes and even cancer, with detox diets. The long-term costs of these approaches can be severe and are based on a potential delay of treatment and may therefore involve the financial burden of intensive clinical therapy as well as the long-term suffering of physical harm.

HOW TO MAKE A DETOX DIET WORK FOR YOU

Detox diets result in lower energy levels, and they can cause digestive issues, so don't try these plans if you're going to be traveling, competing, and so forth.

Keep your motivation in mind. If you're detoxing to break from bad habits or identify food allergies, you've got a valiant reason to go through the arduous exercise of saying "no, thank you" again and again.

Detox diets should only be followed for short bursts of time, so if you're looking for a long-term solution to whatever ails you, look elsewhere.

Plan ahead. There's a good chance your next business lunch won't offer lemon juice mixed with cayenne pepper or the grain-free, dairy-free, legume-free, sugar-free side dish you've come to love. Make sure you're packing whatever's "allowed" on your plan.

Find a support system. Detox diets are often uncomfortable and unsustainable. You're more likely to stick with it if you have an ally.

What to Eat
& When to Eat It

We all have go-to foods, whether it's a favorite or just what feels familiar. Commit to seeking out new foods and flavors so you can have more diversity in your daily diet. Plan ahead so you can be intentional about making healthy choices and fueling your workouts.

Essential Everyday Foods

Every choice, every bite, makes you. So make it count. Fill your basket, your pantry, your plate with foods that move you toward your goals rather than hamper your efforts. Not sure where to even start? The following tables list a small smattering of can't-lose choices that should always be kept at the ready. I've included the benefits they provide as well as the nutritional info. You can rely on this info as you track your intake. Use it to populate the nutrition facts in your food journal.

Be proud of what's on your plate.

Grains & Carbs

Best consumed raw, whole, and minimally processed. Baked goods, pastas, and other ready-to-eat foods are typically more processed and less nutritious.

Amaranth

Packs a lively, peppery taste and a high level of protein. A single serving is an excellent source of calcium and iron.

serving	½ cup, dry
calories	358
protein	13 g
fat	7 g
carbs	63 g
fiber	7 g

Brown rice

(Or red, black, purple varieties) With five times more fiber than white rice, whole-grain brown rice is well tolerated and easy to digest.

serving	½ cup, dry
calories	320
protein	9 g
fat	3 g
carbs	70 g
fiber	5 g

Buckwheat

Not technically a grain but a cousin to rhubarb, it's commonly found toasted and/or cracked (i.e., kasha).

serving	½ cup, dry
calories	284
protein	10 g
fat	2 g
carbs	62 g
fiber	9 g

Corn

Enjoyed worldwide, whole-grain corn offers more vitamin A than any other grain while also being high in antioxidants and the carotenoids lutein and zeaxanthin.

serving	½ cup, fresh kernels
calories	60
protein	1 g
fat	1 g
carbs	13 g
fiber	2 g

Lentils

Rich in B vitamins, a single serving contains 500 mg of folate, one-third the daily value of potassium, and nearly half your daily zinc needs.

serving	½ cup, dry
calories	330
protein	25 g
fat	1 g
carbs	56 g
fiber	22 g

Millet

The staple grain from India, also commonly eaten in Asia, is incredibly versatile—used in flatbreads, porridges, side dishes, and more.

serving	½ cup, dry
calories	378
protein	11 g
fat	4 g
carbs	73 g
fiber	9 g

GLUTEN FREE

Oats

Oats are almost always a whole grain since they rarely have their bran and germ removed in processing. The fiber in oats, beta-glucan, is effective at lowering cholesterol.

serving	½ cup, dry
calories	300
protein	10 g
fat	5 g
carbs	54 g
fiber	8 g

Quinoa

Available in a variety of colors, this fluffy, filling grain offers a plant-based source of complete protein.

serving	½ cup, dry
calories	313
protein	12 g
fat	5 g
carbs	55 g
fiber	6 g

Sorghum

This ancient grain is usually consumed with its outer layers, meaning it retains the majority of its nutrients. It's also grown from traditional hybrid seeds, making it non-GMO.

serving	½ cup, dry
calories	316
protein	10 g
fat	3 g
carbs	69 g
fiber	6 g

Spelt

Spelt is higher in protein than common wheat. Some who are sensitive to wheat (i.e., not celiac) report that they can tolerate spelt, but this is anecdotal.

serving	½ cup, dry
calories	294
protein	13 g
fat	2 g
carbs	61 g
fiber	10 g

Sweet potato

An excellent choice for an easy-to-digest carb packed with antioxidants, like vitamin A.

serving	½ cup, cubed
calories	57
protein	1 g
fat	0 g
carbs	13 g
fiber	2 g

Whole wheat

Includes varieties like spelt, kamut, farro, and durum and products like bulgur and semolina. Wheat is a staple fuel for active individuals and offers a host of essential nutrients.

serving	½ cup, flour
calories	204
protein	8 g
fat	2 g
carbs	43 g
fiber	7 g

Resource: For more information on the history and benefits of carb sources like some of these, visit Oldways Whole Grains Council at wholegrainscouncil.org.

Vegetables

These nutritional powerhouses should always find a way onto your plate. Look for seasonal fresh produce or nutrient-dense frozen versions.

Beet

Summer, fall, winter

Prized for its ability to improve vasodilation (blood flow) as well as performance in some athletes.

serving	2, 2-inch beets
calories	71
protein	3 g
fat	0 g
carbs	16 g
fiber	5 g

Bell pepper

Summer, fall

Rich in vitamin C, a nutrient that assists in the production of collagen, leading to prevention of bruises and proper wound healing.

serving	1 cup, chopped
calories	30
protein	1 g
fat	0 g
carbs	7 g
fiber	3 g

Broccoli

Spring

Rich in vitamin C, combine broccoli with foods rich in iron to enhance the body's ability to absorb iron.

serving	1 cup, fresh
calories	31
protein	3 g
fat	0 g
carbs	6 g
fiber	2 g

Brussels sprouts

Fall, winter

Baked, steamed, or lightly sautéed, these mini cabbages are as rich in nutrients as they are in flavor.

serving	1 cup, fresh
calories	38
protein	3 g
fat	0 g
carbs	8 g
fiber	3 g

Carrot

Year-round

Rich in vitamin A and beta-carotene, nutrients that are essential for healthy vision, immune function, and cell membrane integrity.

serving	2 med. or 14 baby
calories	50
protein	2 g
fat	0 g
carbs	12 g
fiber	4 g

Cauliflower

Fall

Mild and hearty, this vegetable is a great substitute for starchy potatoes and can be mashed, puréed, or riced.

serving	1 cup, fresh
calories	27
protein	2 g
fat	0 g
carbs	5 g
fiber	2 g

Cucumber

Summer

Contains water and electrolytes. Serve sliced with dip as a healthy alternative to a side of chips.

serving	1 cup, sliced
calories	16
protein	1 g
fat	0 g
carbs	4 g
fiber	1 g

Kale

Spring, fall, winter

This versatile member of the cabbage family is best enjoyed in a salad, a sautéed side dish, or in your favorite smoothie.

serving	1 cup, chopped
calories	8
protein	1 g
fat	0 g
carbs	1 g
fiber	1 g

Mushrooms

Spring, fall

Rich in selenium, a trace mineral responsible for immune function, healthy thyroid function, and protection of vitamin E stores.

serving	1 cup, chopped
calories	19
protein	2 g
fat	0 g
carbs	3 g
fiber	1 g

Pumpkin

Fall

A serving provides well over 200% RDA for vitamin A, protecting vision and essential for cell differentiation.

serving	1 cup, canned
calories	83
protein	3 g
fat	1 g
carbs	20 g
fiber	7 g

Spinach

Spring, fall

Plant source of lutein, a carotenoid that plays a role in vision as well as cognition.

serving	1 cup, chopped
calories	7
protein	1 g
fat	0 g
carbs	1 g
fiber	1 g

Tomatoes

Summer

Rich in lycopene, a phytonutrient that plays a role in the fight against cancers such as prostate and skin. Also offers many cardiovascular benefits.

serving	1 cup, chopped
calories	32
protein	2 g
fat	0 g
carbs	7 g
fiber	2 g

Fruit

A great source of vitamins and carbohydrates, fiber-rich fruit can be enjoyed fresh in season or frozen any time of the year in a smoothie, a parfait, or some other creative dish.

Apple

Year-round

With so many varieties, find a favorite and enjoy a fresh apple daily while boosting your fiber and vitamin intake.

serving	1 medium
calories	95
protein	0 g
fat	0 g
carbs	25 g
fiber	4 g

Banana

Year-round

A common go-to for energy, bananas are quick to digest and contain potassium, helpful for proper muscle function.

serving	1 medium
calories	105
protein	1 g
fat	0 g
carbs	27 g
fiber	3 g

Blackberries

Summer

Rich in antioxidants while being high in fiber and thus low in net carb content, berries are a great choice for a filling, low-cal sweet treat.

serving	1 cup
calories	62
protein	2 g
fat	1 g
carbs	14 g
fiber	7 g

Blueberries

Summer

Recent research suggests that a diet rich in blueberries may be linked to improvements in brain health.

serving	1 cup
calories	84
protein	1 g
fat	0 g
carbs	21 g
fiber	4 g

Citrus

Spring, winter

(Lemons, limes, oranges) Rich in vitamin C, a nutrient that assists in the production of collagen, a component of all connective tissues (tendons, teeth, bone, ligaments).

serving	1 medium fruit
calories	69
protein	1 g
fat	0 g
carbs	17 g
fiber	4 g

Cranberries

Fall

Packed with PACS (proanthocyanidins), phytochemicals that thwart bacteria's ability to adhere to tissues. Daily intake is proven to ward off ulcers, dental cavities, and UTIs.

serving	¼ cup dried
calories	106
protein	0 g
fat	0 g
carbs	27 g
fiber	2 g

Dates and figs

Fall

A source of easy-to-digest carbs and a natural alternative for foodies looking to fuel mid-workout.

serving	2 Medjool dates
calories	110
protein	1 g
fat	0 g
carbs	31 g
fiber	3 g

Melon

Summer

(Includes watermelon, honeydew, canteloupe) A great, refreshing choice thanks to its high water content.

serving	1 cup, cubed
calories	46
protein	1 g
fat	0 g
carbs	11 g
fiber	1 g

Pomegranate

Fall

Provides nearly half your daily fiber needs. Enjoy arils (the seeds) as a topping on salads, cereals, or yogurt.

serving	1 4-inch fruit
calories	234
protein	5 g
fat	3 g
carbs	53 g
fiber	11 g

Stone fruit

Summer

(Plums, apricots, peaches, nectarines) The colorful skin of these fruits is a reminder of their high antioxidant and phytonutrient content.

serving	1 fruit (plum)
calories	118
protein	1 g
fat	0 g
carbs	31 g
fiber	6 g

Strawberries

Spring, summer

Rely on this source of vitamin C to support your immune function during times of heavy training.

serving	1 cup
calories	46
protein	1 g
fat	0 g
carbs	11 g
fiber	3 g

Tart cherries

Summer

Shown to decrease inflammation, exercise-induced muscle pain, and other symptoms of muscle damage. Choose minimally processed juice (in a light-shielding bottle) or frozen. Use during times of heavy training.

serving	1 cup juice
calories	130
protein	1 g
fat	0 g
carbs	32 g
fiber	0 g

Resource: For more information on the seasonality of produce, check out the Seasonality Charts from Center for Urban Education about Sustainable Agriculture, available at cuesa.org.

Fat

Rich in essential fatty acids, energy-dense fats and oils help your body absorb nutrients found in other foods. Choose a variety throughout the day.

Almonds

A good source of biotin, which is essential for healthy protein, carb, and fat metabolism.

serving	1 oz.
calories	170
protein	6 g
fat	15 g
carbs	6 g
fiber	3 g

Avocado

A plant source of vitamin E, which is a strong antioxidant and a promoter of healthy immune function.

serving	½ avocado
calories	114
protein	1 g
fat	10 g
carbs	6 g
fiber	5 g

Butter

Once avoided due to its saturated fat content, full-fat butter is finally having its day in the sun. (Avoid margarines, which are heavily processed and contain trans fats.)

serving	1 Tbsp.
calories	102
protein	0 g
fat	12 g
carbs	0 g
fiber	0 g

Canola oil

Sometimes avoided due to GMO content, canola oil is actually one of the best heart-healthy plant oils. Its mild flavor and high smoke point make it a chef's favorite.

serving	1 Tbsp.
calories	124
protein	0 g
fat	14 g
carbs	0 g
fiber	0 g

Chia seeds

Viscous and filling when put in water, these seeds are rich in omega-3s and an egg-substitue for vegans.

serving	1 Tbsp.
calories	50
protein	2 g
fat	3 g
carbs	4 g
fiber	3 g

Coconut oil

A common source of MCTs, coconut oil is shelf-stable and versatile, thanks to its high saturated fat content and high smoke point.

serving	1 Tbsp.
calories	121
protein	0 g
fat	13 g
carbs	0 g
fiber	0 g

Flax seeds

A powerful source of inflammation-fighting omega-3s. (Must be ground to be digestible.)

serving	1 Tbsp.
calories	37
protein	1 g
fat	3 g
carbs	2 g
fiber	2 g

MCT oil

Medium-chain triglycerides are absorbed rapidly and converted to energy rather than being stored in fat tissue.

serving	1 Tbsp.
calories	115
protein	0 g
fat	14 g
carbs	0 g
fiber	0 g

Nut butters

(Peanut, almond, cashew, hazelnut) Natural nut butters have no added sugars or hydrogenated oils, which is helpful in your quest for health.

serving	1 Tbsp. natural peanut butter
calories	96
protein	4 g
fat	8 g
carbs	4 g
fiber	1 g

Olive oil

Best used in dressings and finishing oils. High heat can cause pure EVOO varieties to burn and smoke.

serving	1 Tbsp.
calories	119
protein	0 g
fat	14 g
carbs	0 g
fiber	0 g

Pistachios

Ounce for ounce, this nut offers the most kernals per portion. Pistachios in the shell provide a visual reminder of the portion you've enjoyed.

serving	1 oz.
calories	162
protein	6 g
fat	13 g
carbs	8 g
fiber	3 g

Walnuts

Rich in manganese and magnesium, two minerals that are essential in the formation of healthy bone and cartilage.

serving	1 oz.
calories	185
protein	4 g
fat	18 g
carbs	4 g
fiber	2 g

Protein

Providing a variety of essential amino acids, organic and sustainable proteins play an important role in every snack and meal.

Animal Protein

Beef, grass-fed

Lean cuts are packed with protein and offer omega-3 fatty acids.

serving	3 oz. grilled (strip steak)
calories	100
protein	20 g
fat	2 g
carbs	0 g
fiber	0 g

Eggs

Rich in nutrients like choline and lutein, which are hard to get elsewhere.

serving	1, large
calories	78
protein	6 g
fat	5 g
carbs	1 g
fiber	0 g

Pork

Lean cuts like loin and tenderloin are your best bets.

serving	3 oz. grilled (tenderloin)
calories	122
protein	22 g
fat	3 g
carbs	0 g
fiber	0 g

Poultry, skinless

Enjoy both white and dark meat.

serving	3 oz. grilled (chicken breast)
calories	128
protein	26 g
fat	3 g
carbs	0 g
fiber	0 g

Salmon, wild-caught

Rich in flavor and omega-3 fatty acids.

serving	3 oz. baked
calories	155
protein	22 g
fat	7 g
carbs	0 g
fiber	0 g

Tuna

Canned or fresh, tuna is an excellent source of readily available, high-quality protein.

serving	3 oz. canned in water
calories	90
protein	20 g
fat	1 g
carbs	0 g
fiber	0 g

Dairy & Dairy Alternative Protein

Cheese

Packed with nutrients (and fat and calories), a serving is the size of about four small cubes.

serving	1 oz. (cheddar)
calories	115
protein	6 g
fat	9 g
carbs	1 g
fiber	0 g

Cottage cheese, low-fat

Packed with casein, this protein is slow to digest, supplying the body with a stream of amino acids for hours.

serving	1 cup
calories	92
protein	12 g
fat	3 g
carbs	5 g
fiber	0 g

Greek yogurt, plain, low-fat

A protein and nutrition powerhouse. Enjoy as a stand-alone snack or use in cooking in place of sour cream or higher-fat dairy options.

serving	5.3 oz.
calories	146
protein	20 g
fat	4 g
carbs	8 g
fiber	0 g

Kefir milk, plain, low-fat

A fermented dairy drink that offers protein, calcium, and beneficial probiotics. Look for an unsweetened version to avoid added sugar.

serving	1 cup
calories	110
protein	10 g
fat	2 g
carbs	12 g
fiber	0 g

Milk, 1%

Rich in calcium, vitamin D, and protein. Use 1% if cutting calories and 2% for a creamy lower-fat alternative to whole milk.

serving	1 cup
calories	102
protein	8 g
fat	2 g
carbs	12 g
fiber	0 g

Nut "milks"

Choices range from almond and cashew to oat and pea. Look for no sugar added and fortified with calcium and vitamin D.

serving	1 cup unsweetened almond milk
calories	39
protein	2 g
fat	3 g
carbs	2 g
fiber	0 g

Legume Protein

Black beans

A good source of protein, fiber, and folate.

serving	½ cup, boiled
calories	114
protein	8 g
fat	0 g
carbs	20 g
fiber	7 g

Chickpeas

(Also called garbanzo beans) These are versatile and rich in protein and fiber.

serving	½ cup, canned
calories	106
protein	6 g
fat	2 g
carbs	16 g
fiber	5 g

Lentils

Dry lentils are inexpensive, easy to cook, and can provide a nutrient boost to soups, stews, and other dishes.

serving	½ cup, boiled
calories	115
protein	9 g
fat	0 g
carbs	20 g
fiber	8 g

Peanuts

A popular "nut," these legumes are rich in B vitamins and trace minerals, such as copper, manganese, and selenium.

serving	35 peanuts
calories	160
protein	7 g
fat	14 g
carbs	4 g
fiber	2 g

Peas

Easy to add to soups and stews and commonly found in plant protein powders.

serving	½ cup, boiled
calories	116
protein	8 g
fat	0 g
carbs	21 g
fiber	8 g

Soybeans, edamame, tofu

One of the few plant proteins containing adequate amounts of essential amino acids.

serving	½ cup
calories	94
protein	9 g
fat	4 g
carbs	7 g
fiber	4 g

Pre-Workout Fuel

To decide whether or not to eat before a workout, consider your goals. To get lean and mean, you may want to train on empty, drawing on the fuel stores you have in place, and nutritionally recover (i.e., eat) once you're done. If you're looking to *own* the workout or PR at an event, fuel ahead of time so your system is primed for performance. In either scenario, your success hinges upon nutrient timing, quantity, and quality.

 Casual workout or looking to get lean? Deplete before you eat.
Intense workout or looking to PR? Eat before you compete.

Two to Three Hours Before a Workout

Avoid indulgent, heavy items as they take longer to digest. Same goes for protein—pace your intake throughout your day. Digestion takes energy, and you want to direct that energy toward your muscles. Great choices in the hours before a workout include a cup of pasta tossed with some marinara sauce and a cup of skim milk. Or try a turkey sandwich, hold the mayo and go easy on that 15-gram fiber bread. Plan to meet your fiber and micronutrient needs post-workout.

If you're looking to go long or to PR (and are willing to get technical), consume a half gram of carbs per pound of body weight for each hour that you have before showtime. In other words, if you have two hours before your race starts and you weigh 150 pounds, consume 150 grams of carbs (150 × 0.5 × 2) in order to be primed to tackle the challenge in front of you!

Goal: Eat enough, but don't stuff yourself. Save high-fat, high-fiber, and spicy foods for after the workout. Prioritize fluids, including electrolyte-rich beverages, for optimal hydration. If your workout will be longer than 90 minutes, some of your pre-workout fluid can come from carb-rich sports drinks since you'll need the quick-burning fuel.

30 to 60 Minutes Before an Intense Workout or Competition

Grab carbs with a touch of protein and sip on fluids so you show up hydrated. Good options include oatmeal with fruit, low-fat yogurt topped with fruit and granola, cereal (try to avoid high-fiber cereals like bran flakes), or a bagel topped with a scrambled egg and some fruit.

Goal: Before your workouts, top off the tank with just enough fuel to quiet your hunger and your thirst. Your GI system will derail your workout if you overdo it. For workouts or races lasting longer than 90 minutes, pack some mid-workout fuel to keep you going.

Pre-Workout Snacks and Small Meal Ideas

Here is a variety of healthy choices to better fuel your workouts.

1 medium fresh fruit with 2 Tbsp. nut butter

The potassium and fluid in the fruit helps maintain hydration status, while the nut butter offers heart-healthy fat and energy.

calories 290
protein 8 g
fat 17 g
carbs 32 g
fiber 6 g

1 cup low-fiber cereal with ½ cup skim milk

Fuel up with some easy-to-digest carbs and a bit of protein for steady energy.

calories 155
protein 6 g
fat 1 g
carbs 13 g
fiber <1 g

Bagel half with 1 Tbsp. nut butter & 1 Tbsp. jam or honey

A blend of carbohydrates and nutrients for both quick and long-lasting energy.

calories 300
protein 9 g
fat 9 g
carbs 50 g
fiber 2 g

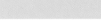

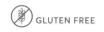

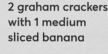

2 fig cookies

Easily digested and packed with high-energy carbs and extra vitamins and minerals.

calories	220
protein	4 g
fat	5 g
carbs	40 g
fiber	4 g

½ cup mixed fruit with ½ cup 2% milk-fat cottage cheese

Offers vitamins and minerals such as calcium, potassium, and vitamin D. The casein protein in cottage cheese will fuel your muscles long after your workout.

calories	150
protein	12 g
fat	3 g
carbs	20 g
fiber	1 g

2 graham crackers with 1 medium sliced banana

Packed with carbs to top off glycogen stores, this easy-to-digest choice is perfect before a tempo workout or HIIT session.

calories	245
protein	3 g
fat	4 g
carbs	50 g
fiber	4 g

½ cup dry steel-cut oats prepared with 1 cup skim milk

Rich in fiber to keep you full and B vitamins to support energy and metabolism, this is an excellent choice any time of the day.

calories	405
protein	20 g
fat	6 g
carbs	64 g
fiber	10 g

1 cup plain yogurt topped with 1 Tbsp. chopped pecans & 1 Tbsp. dried fruit pieces

Rich in potassium, calcium, and magnesium, this simple snack aids in muscle performance and supports bone health.

calories	230
protein	14 g
fat	9 g
carbs	25 g
fiber	1 g

1 cup berries with 6 oz. plain Greek yogurt & ¼ cup homemade granola

Satiating protein, nutrients (calcium, vitamin D, and potassium) and various antioxidants to support immune function.

calories	280
protein	20 g
fat	5 g
carbs	42 g
fiber	7 g

Pre-Workout Snacks and Small Meal Ideas *(continued)*

1 small whole wheat pita, 10 baby carrots & 2 Tbsp. hummus

Savory option offers a boost of iron and electrolytes.

calories	225
protein	10 g
fat	5 g
carbs	40 g
fiber	9 g

2 waffles with 2 Tbsp. maple syrup

The source of energy in maple syrup (primarily sucrose) fuels your system with a blend of glucose and fructose. This mix of sugar sources allows more grams of glycogen-restoring fuel to be absorbed without GI upset.

calories	285
protein	5 g
fat	6 g
carbs	56 g
fiber	1 g

2 slices whole-grain bread, 1 medium banana & 1 Tbsp. peanut butter

A blend of fat, protein, and carbs to supply long-lasting energy, vitamins, and minerals. A great choice to fuel a long workout.

calories	340
protein	12 g
fat	11 g
carbs	53 g
fiber	8 g

15 whole-grain crackers topped with 2 Tbsp. nut butter

Easy-to-digest, long-lasting energy.

calories	365
protein	9 g
fat	25 g
carbs	30 g
fiber	5 g

1 cup of Apple Cinnamon O's with 1 cup of skim milk & 1 medium sliced banana

Easy-to-digest, filling choice that is perfect if you have an hour or two to spare but don't want to get too hungry.

calories	345
protein	13 g
fat	3 g
carbs	71 g
fiber	6 g

3 oz. sliced rotisserie chicken with 1 slice whole wheat bread & 1 apple

Long-lasting energy with extra protein to proactively aid in muscle recovery.

calories	350
protein	29 g
fat	5 g
carbs	49 g
fiber	6 g

Mid-Workout Fuel

Intense, long, and critical workouts require a lot of your body. You need to keep gas in your tank if you want it to keep firing on all cylinders. So anytime you're logging a workout lasting longer than 90 minutes, plan for mid-workout fueling. Shorter workouts don't necessarily require a mid-run fuel stop because most of us have enough energy reserves on board to survive anything less than 90 minutes. But on the occasion that you're working out for shorter periods of time and you've either skimped on last night's dinner or you feel run-down and short on energy, there's no harm to adding in mid-run fuel.

How much do you need? Research has found that an intake of 30 to 60 grams of carbs every hour will restock your glycogen and fend off hitting the wall. Athletes going really long (3+ hours) may find benefit in bumping their fuel intake up to 90 grams of carbohydrates, but most of the athletes I've worked with over the years find that an intake of 45 to 60 grams of carbs per hour sufficiently meets their needs. (To determine your hourly fluid needs, see p. 101.)

Find this fuel in sports nutrition gels, chews, bars, and drinks. These items have quick-digesting carbohydrates—a source of glucose mixed with a source of fructose is typically best—along with sodium, chloride, potassium, and other electrolytes. If you prefer solid food choices, grab a snack that sits well in your stomach and is made up of easy-to-digest carbs, minimal protein, minimal fat, and a handful of electrolytes. Many athletes experiment with choices such as raisins, pretzels, their kid's baby food pouches, or even mashed sweet potato (place in a zippered baggie and take it on the go). Be sure to chase your chosen fuel with 4 to 8 ounces of water (most products will offer you advice—check the label).

Add this fuel in within 45 minutes of starting your workout. No need to wait until you're feeling run down. By then you'll have depleted much of your glycogen stores and you'll spend the next few miles trying to play catch-up (never a pretty sight). Instead, fuel early, fuel often, include water to stay hydrated, and fuel in small increments. Sports nutrition products are concentrated sources of fuel, and this glob of energy will sit in your gut and be slow to absorb unless you dilute it—so don't skimp on water and never chase a gel with sports drink. Try taking a few chews or half a gel at a time and evenly spread those 30 to 60 grams of carbs out over the hour. Experiment with brands, flavors, forms, and amounts until you find the one that works for you. Write down your trial and error in your journal so you know what does and, perhaps more important, doesn't work for you. When you find the mix that leaves you feeling energized and never sick to your stomach or running for the bathroom, stick with it for the long run and on race day.

Fuel for Recovery

It's always important to eat *after* a workout. All workouts demand some degree of nutritional recovery, and the more intense the workout, the more serious the recovery. Skip this critical step and you'll have difficulty making progress because you'll be worn down, sore, and less motivated to move. Similar to the how and the why of fueling *before* a workout, the quantity and choices of food consumed post-workout depend on your goals.

> **Looking to get lean and mean?** Recover with adequate protein to repair and restore.
>
> **Looking to perform and PR?** Repair with protein and restock with carbs in preparation for tomorrow's training session.
>
> **Want the best of both worlds?** Repair and recover with adequate protein and a hint of carbs (preparing you for later workouts), but flex your willpower to avoid refilling the tank and then some!

30 to 60 Minutes After a Workout

Refuel within an hour of workout completion, keeping in mind that the fitter you are, the quicker you need to recover. The timing of your next workout also plays into the recovery equation—the sooner your next session, the sooner you should refuel. It's during this 30- to-60-minute window that your muscles are primed to take in nutrients and glycogen. When you nutritionally recover, your system stops breaking down and instead rebuilds from the stress you just put it through. A properly designed recovery meal or snack prevents further muscle breakdown, helps optimize muscle and liver glycogen stores, and ultimately promotes desired adaptations to training, helping you build fitness.

Plan your recovery to make your nutrition goals a reality. Cutting calories? Then skip the recovery snack and instead design a quick post-workout *meal* to contain the protein and fluids you need.

Lean & Mean Recovery: 15–30 g protein, plus fluids to rehydrate.
Performance Recovery: 15–30 g protein, plus two to four times as much carbs plus fluids to rehydrate.

Push yourself. Prioritize recovery. Performance will follow.

Recovery Snacks and Meals

All of these options contain 15 to 40 grams of protein with varying amounts of carbohydrates.

Smoothie with 1 cup unsweetened nut milk, 1 scoop vegan protein powder (15 g protein), 1 serving of fresh fruit, 1 cup ice

Fresh fruit and milk help recover fluid losses while also providing vitamins and minerals and all-important protein.

calories	250
protein	26 g
fat	4 g
carbs	30 g
fiber	7 g

2 hard-boiled eggs, 1 mozzarella cheese stick, 1 oz. beef jerky, 10 baby carrots

This snack provides nearly 100% of your daily vitamin C, a powerful antioxidant that works to keep you healthy when mileage is high.

calories	310
protein	24 g
fat	19 g
carbs	13 g
fiber	3 g

1 whole-grain tortilla filled with 1 cup sliced veggies, ¼ cup hummus and 2 Tbsp. crumbled feta

Recover with complex carbs, antioxidants, and a blend of plant protein from grains and legumes.

calories	420
protein	39 g
fat	16 g
carbs	34 g
fiber	8 g

Panini with 2 slices whole wheat bread, 3 oz. chicken breast, 1 slice cheese (2% fat) & extra veggies

High in protein, this choice is best following a tough workout or high-mileage week.

calories	315
protein	37 g
fat	7 g
carbs	26 g
fiber	5 g

1 medium banana spread with 2 Tbsp. peanut butter & ready-to-drink protein shake (30 g protein)

Easy to digest and perfect for on-the-go runners who are short on recovery time.

calories	450
protein	38 g
fat	20 g
carbs	35 g
fiber	7 g

Fried egg on 1 toasted whole wheat English muffin with 1¼ cups fresh blueberries, 5 oz. plain Greek yogurt

Balanced with protein and fiber to keep you full as you recover after a hard effort.

calories	362
protein	27 g
fat	6 g
carbs	50 g
fiber	7 g

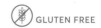
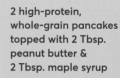

½ cup raw oats cooked with 1 cup skim milk and 1 scoop protein powder (15 g whey protein), topped with 1 sliced banana & 2 Tbsp. dried cranberries

Easy on the stomach after a hard workout, this snack offers whey protein to rebuild and oat-based carbs to restock.

calories	535
protein	29 g
fat	5 g
carbs	91 g
fiber	5 g

Smoothie with 2 scoops protein powder (30 g protein per serving), 1 Tbsp. powdered peanut butter, 1 Tbsp. cocoa, 1 cup of skim milk & ice

Low in fat but high in calcium, potassium, carbs, and protein. Easy on the stomach and great for rehydrating.

calories	275
protein	39 g
fat	5 g
carbs	21 g
fiber	4 g

2 high-protein, whole-grain pancakes topped with 2 Tbsp. peanut butter & 2 Tbsp. maple syrup

Maple syrup is packed with natural antioxidants, polyphenols, vitamins, and minerals. 2 Tbsp. also provides over half your daily value of manganese.

calories	475
protein	15 g
fat	17 g
carbs	69 g
fiber	6 g

1 cup brown rice, 1 cup shredded pork loin, 1 cup steamed veggies

This simple dish effectively restocks, repairs, replaces lost nutrients, and gives you a boost of fiber.

calories	350
protein	18 g
fat	6 g
carbs	57 g
fiber	5 g

3 cups spring mix topped with 2 oz. fresh goat cheese, ½ cup chopped chicken breast & 2 Tbsp. Italian vinaigrette

Cut calories without neglecting recovery with this recovery "meal" to be enjoyed within an hour post-workout.

calories	360
protein	35 g
fat	20 g
carbs	8 g
fiber	2 g

1 cup sliced raw vegetables, ¼ cup hummus, 1 oz. low-fat cheddar, 1 oz. crumbled goat cheese

With nearly 40% of daily value for phosphorus and 20% of calcium and magnesium, this snack is a great choice for athletes looking for better bone health.

calories	245
protein	18 g
fat	15 g
carbs	13 g
fiber	6 g

Hydrate for better recovery

It's common to be dehydrated by the time you finish a sweat session or cross a finish line. Accordingly, it's important to get plenty of fluids ASAP so you can speed recovery. If the session was light or the conditions mild, water will do just fine. But if it was a serious sweat sesh in more extreme weather (hot and humid or cold and dry), reach for some electrolytes too. Only when water is consumed along with food or drink containing sodium, chloride, and other minerals will the fluid be retained in your system and effectively restore your hydration balance. If you want to be sure you've recovered the fluid you lost, weigh yourself before and after the activity. Determine how many ounces were lost during the event, and drink as much—and then some—until you recover the lost weight. Or you can simply drink until your thirst diminishes and your urine returns to a light straw color. Try out these options to fuel your workouts and promote recovery.

<1 HOUR WORKOUT

16 oz. water + 1 packet/tablet hypotonic solution (e.g., Pedialyte®)

Replace salt losses at a concentration designed to move quickly from your gut to surrounding tissues—in other words, no gut bomb!

calories	25
protein	0 g
fat	0 g
carbs	6 g
sodium	240 mg
potassium	180 mg
chloride	290 mg
fiber	2 mg

1+ HOUR WORKOUT

16 oz. water, 1 serving 2–6% carbohydrate solution with adequate sodium and potassium

Meet your fluid, electrolyte, and energy needs so you can keep pushing the pace.

calories	115 or less
protein	0–1 g
fat	0 g
carbs	10–28 g
sodium	230–650 mg
potassium	80–200 mg
chloride	0–115 mg
fiber	0–40 mg

POST-WORKOUT

1–2 scoops whey protein, 1 cup milk, 1 cup ice, 1 cup frozen berries + 1 banana

Aim to get carbs (0.5 g carbs/lb.) and protein (15–30 g) within an hour of finishing.

calories	425
protein	30 g
fat	7 g
carbs	59 g
fiber	6 g

Balance Your Macros, Hunger & Mood

2

Set Your Nutrition Goals

Tell someone, anyone, that you're a registered dietitian and it's as if you have opened the floodgates for an impromptu Q&A session. Without fail, the barrage of rapid-fire questions always includes this one: "How many calories do I need?" As if being an RD gives you the automatic ability to size up a complete stranger in the grocery checkout line and rattle off an accurate number. While, yes, this situation has actually happened, sometimes it feels as if throwing out a guess might be about as accurate as some of the calorie calculators out there. You've likely encountered these tools on apps or websites, so you know the drill: Input your gender, age, and weight, and it will spit out your calorie needs. If only our calorie needs could be so simple as a triangulation of gender, weight, and age. In truth, energy needs are complex and flux from day to day, month to month, until infinity. The amount of food you need to eat to lose, maintain, or gain weight is based on the following factors:

▷ Resting metabolic rate (the energy needed to keep all systems going at rest), typically 60–80 percent of daily energy needs
▷ Thermic effect of food (the energy needed to digest food), typically 10 percent of daily energy needs
▷ Exercise and nonexercise activity (e.g., fidgeting, folding laundry), making up the remainder of your daily energy needs

Note that this last category can range from minimal to vast and can vary widely from person to person.

The best way to determine your energy needs is in a lab setting, using a dual-energy X-ray absorptiometry (DEXA) scan for body composition measurements and an indirect calorimetry machine for resting metabolic rate measurements. These tests are available at some university nutrition clinics or exercise physiology labs, and in some hospitals. By making an appointment and getting scanned or having your resting metabolic rate tested rather than estimated, you'll confidently be able to determine the level of calories needed to fuel your day.

Unfortunately, this gold standard of measurement isn't available to most of us, and equations like the one listed on the following page were created to estimate daily needs. Just remember, these equations result in an *estimate*—a number that will evolve over time. So grab a pencil and a calculator and let's get started.

Decide Your Goal Weight

First, think about the number you'd like to see on the scale. While health is about *so much more* than that damn number on the scale, that number does serve as a starting point. Now, you may be wondering if your goal weight is realistic or healthy. To answer this question for clients, I take into account body mass index, ideal body weight, and feel-good weight.

Body mass index is a weight-to-height ratio used to classify weight status. It has its limitations, such as overestimating body fat in muscular athletes and underestimating body fat in those who have lost muscle mass, but it's generally useful as a baseline for weight and obesity, and it's a good gauge of risk for diseases that can occur as body fat percentage increases. In general populations (i.e., not athletes), higher BMIs can be correlated with higher risk of certain diseases, such as heart disease, high blood pressure, type 2 diabetes, gallstones, breathing problems, and certain cancers.

Body mass index is calculated by dividing weight in kilograms by height in square meters (kg/m²). If you prefer English measurements, the equation for BMI is as follows:

$$\frac{\text{weight in pounds} \times 703}{(\text{height in inches} \times \text{height in inches})} = \text{BMI}$$

What does that mean? Are you at a healthy BMI, or do you have some work to do? BMI is classified into underweight, normal (healthy) weight, overweight, and obese. The categories are as follows:

	Underweight	Normal weight	Overweight	Obese
BMI	<18.5	18.5–24.9	25–29.9	>30

Finally, there's one more gut check when it comes to deciding upon a goal weight. Ask the question: *At what weight do I feel good?* At what weight do you feel energized and ready to tackle your day, do you feel comfortable in your own skin, and are your blood pressure, heart rate, blood glucose, and blood lipid levels right where your doctor wants them to be? When you arrive at this number, compare it to your ideal body weight range, verify that it falls within the range of a healthy BMI, and you'll have a great place to begin.

Determine Your Daily Energy Needs

How many calories you target in a day will vary depending on whether you need to gain, maintain, or lose weight to reach your goal weight. Choose the appropriate path and crunch the numbers to get started.

Determine your ideal body weight

Using the Hamwi method, you can create another point of reference before settling on a goal weight:

(106 + 6 for every inch of height over 5 ft.) +/- 10%

(100 + 5 for every inch of height over 5 ft.) +/- 10%

For example, the ideal body weight of a 6-foot male would be calculated as follows:

(106 + 6[12]) = 178 lb. +/- 10% → 160 to 196 lb.

Current Weight

Feel-Good Weight

Goal Weight

Note: Set a goal that's both healthy and achievable. For most people, weight will fluctuate between 0.5 and 2 pounds per week depending on caloric intake and activity.

➤➤ Goal: Weight Loss

If you want to lose weight, I recommend determining your resting metabolic rate (RMR) and aiming to hit this number as a starting point. Your RMR is essentially the number of calories you need each day to keep your vital organs functioning, your brain thinking, your heart pumping, and so on. It's typically not a high number because it's the bare minimum number of calories your body needs at rest. Many experts suggest that by targeting a calorie intake right around your RMR and adding in some strength work to protect muscle, weight loss will occur at a rate that won't negatively impact your metabolism and you'll swap fat mass for muscle mass.

Your RMR represents about 60 to 80 percent of your total energy expenditure if you're sedentary—thankfully, you've already bought in to not being sedentary. **There's a wide range of how many calories you might need to add to this RMR to fuel your day if you are working out regularly.** Research finds that RMR alone may account for just 34 to 42 percent of total caloric needs in elite endurance athletes.

If you want to lose weight, and you're not ready to ramp up your workouts quite yet, your RMR is the number you should start with. If you're fairly active yet want to lose weight, begin with your RMR and add in some calories to cover some (not all) of your exercise. If you want to maintain or gain weight, you have a little more math to do.

➤ Goal: Weight Maintenance

If you're looking to maintain weight, you'll need to take both your RMR and your level of physical activity into account in order to figure out your daily calorie needs.

Think about what your day looks like. The more active you are, the more energy you need to consume to fuel this activity while also maintaining your weight. Here are some questions to help you identify your activity factor:

Do you spend most of your day sitting and are fairly sedentary? If so, we need to talk, but until then, **multiply by activity factor of 1.1.**

RMR ×1.1
Activity Factor

Are you fairly active throughout the day (e.g., activities of daily living plus some walking now and again) but don't participate in purposeful exercise? **Multiply by activity factor of 1.4.**

RMR ×1.4
Activity Factor

How to find your
resting metabolic rate

(using the Mifflin–St. Jeor equation)

1

Start with your weight in kilograms: Just divide your weight in pounds by 2.2.

2

Next, convert your height to centimeters: Multiply your height in inches by 2.54.

3

Now, apply this formula:

(10 × weight [kg])

+ (6.25 × height [cm])

– (5 × age [yr]) + 5

= **calories**

(10 × weight [kg])

+ (6.25 × height [cm])

– (5 × age [yr]) – 161

= **calories**

RESTING METABOLIC RATE

Note: Many online RMR calculators use the Harris-Benedict equation to determine RMR. But for many, this equation overestimates daily calorie needs—by as much as 5 percent, which can hamper your efforts to get lean and mean (which is why I use the Mifflin–St. Jeor equation).

Do you break a sweat for 30 minutes a day, a few days a week? **Multiply by activity factor of 1.6.**

RMR ×1.6
Activity Factor

Are you regularly active, logging one hour of exercise a day? **Multiply by activity factor of 1.8.**

RMR ×1.8
Activity Factor

Are you intensely training for race day and logging two to three hours every day? **Multiply by activity factor of 1.9 to 2.2+.**

RMR ×1.9–2.2+
Activity Factor

Note: These activity factors are based on my work with clients and are adapted from guidelines by the National Academy of Medicine.

➤ Goal: Weight Gain

Now, let's say you want to gain weight. You need to take your RMR and your activity into account, but if you want to put on mass, it will take additional substrate to make it happen. This means you need to fuel your day as well as your growth.

Think about what your day looks like. The more active you are, the more energy you'll need to consume in order to fuel this activity while also putting on mass. These questions will help you identify your activity factor:

Do you spend most of your day sitting and are fairly sedentary? Again, we need to talk, but until then, **multiply by activity factor of 1.39.**

RMR ×1.39
Activity Factor

Are you fairly active throughout the day but don't participate in purposeful exercise? **Multiply by activity factor of 1.59.**

RMR ×1.59
Activity Factor

Do you break a sweat for 30 minutes a day, a few days a week? **Multiply by activity factor of 1.75.**

RMR ×1.75
Activity Factor

Are you regularly active, logging 60 minutes of exercise a day? **Multiply by activity factor of 2.**

RMR ×2
Activity Factor

Are you intensely training for race day and logging two to three hours every day? **Multiply by activity factor of 2.5+.**

RMR ×2.5+
Activity Factor

You still with me? Here's an example: A 35-year-old woman weighs 150 pounds. She is 5'7" and wants to maintain her weight; she exercises every other day for 30 minutes.

Weight **150 lb. / 2.2 = 68.2 kg**
Height **5'7" → 67 in. × 2.54 = 170.2 cm**

([10 × 68.2]		[6.25 × 170.2]		[5 × 35])				× 1.6
Weight	+	Height	−	Age	−	**161**	×	Activity Factor
([682]		[1,063.75]		[175])				× 1.6

= 2,256 calories needed to maintain weight and fuel activity

Once you have a target for your daily energy needs, you can map out a plan for your daily macronutrient intake. Take into account a specific diet you are hoping to implement, or find a macro mix that fits your performance, health, and lifestyle goals (see pp. 74–75). Remember to check back in on your energy needs estimate every now and then since it can change based on goals and progress.

Finding Your Macro Mix

Macronutrients play an essential role in facilitating the growth, health, and energy of living organisms. The macros that provide energy throughout the day are carbohydrates, protein, and fat. Throughout this journal, you'll find these nutrients displayed visually in chart form. The real trick is identifying the ratios or distributions of calories that will guide you in your quest for better health, performance, or body composition.

Before you can see what your macro ratio currently looks like, you need to determine your total calorie intake. From there, you can divide your total calories by the calories provided by each nutrient in order to determine the percentage of calories from each source. Then look at the number of grams of carbs, protein, and fat you're consuming. You can find this info on food labels, on an app, or by checking out one of my favorite resources, the USDA FoodData Central (formerly the Food Composition Databases). Multiply each gram by its caloric value: 4 calories per gram for carbohydrates and for protein, 9 calories per gram for energy-dense fat. If you consume alcohol, it's typically not included in a macronutrient distribution. That being said, alcoholic drinks do contain calories and most often these calories come from carbs. So track those drinks (in moderation—right?) by including the calories within your daily total and logging the carbs where they belong. As for those grams of alcohol, at the end of the day, a few grams shouldn't derail your overall macros goal. Include them in your pie chart if it helps you visualize where each and every calorie comes from and where you can make improvements.

So, let's say that you tracked your daily diet in this journal and found out that you consumed 1,800 calories yesterday. After looking at food labels, the Essential Everyday Foods tables on pp. 42–52, and other online sources, you could find out the energy provided by each macro:

CARBS   266 g × 4 calories / gram = 1,064 calories from carbs
PROTEIN 89 g × 4 calories / gram = 356 calories from protein
FAT   42 g × 9 calories / gram = 378 calories from fat

Note: Sometimes food math can get fuzzy; in this example, calories add up to 1,798 calories even though your tracker might say you consumed 1,800. Due to rounding on food labels and in apps. It's close enough.

Now you can determine macronutrient distribution, or the percentage of calories coming from carbs, protein, and fat.

So why does your macronutrient distribution matter? Because even a slight tweaking of the percentages can help you meet your goals. Let's say you follow the 59/20/21 ratio listed above. This is a fairly high percentage of calories from carbohydrates and a moderate amount of protein and fat. If you're an endurance athlete logging some high mileage, this ratio provides enough carbs to fuel those miles, and you're taking in enough protein to protect muscles and enough fat to nourish.

But if circumstances change and your weekly mileage takes a hit, your ratio needs to shift accordingly. Let's say you get injured and your usual cardio routine is shut down for a while. You might need to decrease your calorie goals slightly while sedentary. Since you aren't burning off those energy-providing carbs, any excess intake would be stored as fat anyway. And you likely need more protein to maintain your muscle mass as well as to support healing. So swapping carbs for protein until your workouts pick back up is a solid choice.

Finding Your Macro Mix

Match your macros with your goals

There are specific macronutrient ranges that can be tailored to help you meet your goals, and all of these suggested ranges are backed by multiple research studies. Let's find one that's right for you.

MACRO MIX

- 45–55% carbs
- 20–30% protein
- 20–30% fat

GOAL

Well-balanced approach to healthy eating

Enjoy the flexibility of having all food groups on your plate. You can hit a certain percentage each day or aim to fall somewhere within the listed range. This blend provides variety and room for sustainability, along with a few indulgences. Done right, you'll hit your macros, get focused, and stay on track.

MACRO MIX

- 50–65% carbs
- 20–25% protein
- 15–20% fat

GOAL

Eat for endurance

A higher percentage of carbs can play to your advantage if you are seeking endurance performance. Balance out quick-burning carbs with protein to avoid the risk of getting run-down or injured.

MACRO MIX

- 5–10% carbs
- 15–20% protein
- 70–80% fat

GOAL

Weight loss and/or keto lifestyle

With a very low percentage of calories from carbs, a moderate intake of protein, and a high percentage of calories from fat, this approach demands a controlled approach to carbs. Research shows that higher fat intake coupled with lower carb intake leads to weight loss from fat tissue rather than lean tissue.

Note: The higher the fat and the lower the carbs, the higher the ketones.

MACRO MIX

- 10–25% carbs
- 45–55% protein
- 30–35% fat

GOAL

A low-carb lifestyle

If you find that eating more carbs only leads to cravings and waning energy levels, this macronutrient mix might be a good fit. A low-carb diet works well for anyone who is interested in losing weight and moving toward better health, but is in need of a bit more flexibility in their regular routine.

MACRO MIX

- 40% carbs
- 30% protein
- 30% fat

GOAL

Gain strength, sustain, and recover

Strength and CrossFit athletes, athletes rehabbing an injury, and those looking to tone up can benefit from adequate carbs to fuel their workouts and a fairly even split of calories from protein and fat. This blend is also great for maintaining current weight and also allowing some indulgences but still keeping you focused on your goal of staying toned.

If weight loss and weight maintenance are all about calories in versus calories out, why does your macro mix matter? It's true that you can and will lose weight if you focus solely on calories and consume fewer calories than you burn. But you can also end up "skinny fat," the result of muscle loss coupled with fat retention. What's more, your overall health will suffer if you ignore the macronutrients. Inadequate protein during a calorie deficit will cause you to lose muscle and strength. Inadequate fat intake will negatively impact absorption of essential nutrients as well as many of the hormones that support continued weight loss. And inadequate carbohydrate intake can negatively impact your ability to crank through a calorie-scorching workout.

What if weight loss is not your goal—does the argument that macros matter still stand? Yes! The right macros can help you fend off cravings, keep energy levels steady, and help you see performance improvements at the gym and at the doctor. Sure, you can drop weight by counting calories, but let's not be focused on this metric alone; health in the long run matters more.

The right macro mix will keep you energized and nourished, adequately fuel your workouts, and be sustainable as a lifestyle . . . while also delivering the results you are looking for! To better understand the intricacies and benefits these key macronutrients can deliver, read on.

Carbohydrates

When I was young, I worked in a bagel shop. The line for fat-free, fluffy bagels wrapped around the building, and our only worry was the competition from the bagel and muffin place next door. Those were the days of the "fat is bad, carbs are good" mentality. That same mentality inspired the food industry to promote all-you-can-eat pasta bars and innovate around "fat-free" food claims. Quick pivot to today's world where fat is okay (we think), carbs are mistrusted, and sugar is evil.

While the era of carb as king may have ended, the American diet remains rich in this macronutrient, with the average individual consuming approximately 50 percent of daily calories from carb sources.

The easiest form of calories for your body to convert to energy, carbohydrates are portable, convenient, and inexpensive, but they aren't as satiating as protein or as nourishing as fat. You can eat a whole lotta carbs in no time at all, further fueling the rumor that carbs make you fat. But it's not carbs alone that cause the struggle between you and your skinny jeans. That fight is more complex: It involves total calories, the types of carbs we choose to eat, our emotions, and so much more.

The vast majority of us want and need carbs. We thrive on this energy source and benefit from the foods that naturally provide it, though crackers and candy need not apply. Our health, wellness, and performance goals should determine the type of carbs we consume, the amount, and the timing of intake.

If you are trying to lose weight, let's determine the minimum of carbs needed to fill up the tank without feeling run-down. Then you can spend your calories on harder-working protein and fat.

If you are trying to perform, let's determine the amount needed to adequately fuel your workout and your day so you consistently feel strong and prepared to tackle whatever challenges lie before you.

If you are looking to lose weight *and* perform, your intake will come down to nutrient timing and recovery (see "Fuel for Recovery" on p. 58). In other words, decrease intake slightly but carefully plan your day so you have fuel in the tank before and after your workout. This way, you avoid consuming more carbohydrates than your day demands while also avoiding the risk of depleting your glycogen stores to the point that you can't crank through a workout.

➤➤ How Much Do You Need?

For those of us who really want or need to lose weight or those who are following a low-carb or keto diet for other health benefits, a little carbohydrate goes a long way. But if you have little to spend, every "penny" better work hard for you. When eating a low-carb diet, only nutrient-dense choices that give you a lot of bang for your caloric buck make the cut. If you have more carbs to spend, you have a green light to indulge on occasion, but remember that money is still tight. In other words, if you'd like to lose weight while also training for a half-marathon, you need more carbs and calories than your sedentary friends, but don't follow every workout with heaping plates of carbs. You're unlikely to hit your weight-loss goal. The richest carb consumers are those in heavy training who simply want to fuel their day without shedding any weight. Intense training demands intense fueling so you'll have a pile of cash to spend, but you'll still want to spend it wisely. If you want to start with a general number in mind, consider these options:

> **Looking to lose weight and not ready to ramp up training?** Replace some carbs with protein (you'll likely need to reduce overall intake to hit your calorie goal) and start with 0.5 to 1.3 grams of carbohydrates per pound of body weight.
>
> **Looking to lose weight and are slightly active?** Swap some carbs for satiating protein and aim for a carb intake of 1.3 to 1.75 grams of carbohydrates per pound of body weight.
>
> **Looking to perform and slim down?** Aim for 2 to 2.75 grams of carbohydrates per pound of body weight.
>
> **Looking to fuel your PR?** Get at least 2.5 to 4+ grams of carbs per pound of body weight.

Remember, these guidelines are intended to be a starting point. If you find yourself getting prematurely tired during workouts, up your intake slightly. If you feel energized, but you are not progressing toward your weight goal, take it down a notch, and so on.

There are definitely points in our lives when we truly don't need a lot of carbs as the task at hand doesn't demand this high-octane fuel. In these situations, it's okay to cut back entirely or swap some carbs with protein or fat, depending on your goals. If you're reducing your overall intake of calories, limiting energy-supplying carbs makes more sense than cutting out protein, which plays a host of indispens-able roles in the body, or dietary fat, which offers protection and assists with absorption of nutrients. But rather than eliminate all foods with carbohydrates, take into account other benefits a food has to offer. Cut out crap carbs, but keep the ones that supply essential vitamins, minerals, fiber, and more.

➠ What to Look For

When it comes to making carbs count, your overarching goal is to eat the highest-quality carbs containing the most nutrients with the fewest unhealthy additives. Which is to say that carbs come in two varieties: clean carbs and crap carbs. Fruits, vegetables, dairy, and whole grains are examples of clean carbs, containing the nutrients you need without the junk. These foods offer fiber, antioxidants, and essential vitamins and minerals. Clean carbs deserve to be staples in your diet, no matter what your health, performance, or weight goals may be. Crap carbs do little more than fill your belly, provide you with a quick hit of energy, and then let you down without leaving any nutrients or long-lasting fiber behind. These are the sources of carbs you find in most crackers, cookies, junk food, and so forth. You can cut these calories without negative health repercussions.

Without fail, highly refined grains and sugary treats fit into the crap carb category. A good example of a crap carb is white bread. Sure, it's fortified with some vitamins and minerals (by law), but it's otherwise a vehicle to put deli meat and lettuce into your mouth without getting your hands dirty. It's not that bread is a terrible food. On the contrary! Bread can be delicious and nourishing and full of good-for-you ingredients. But commercial white bread? You know there are better choices out there. There's a huge difference between the refined grains in products such as boxed pastas, bakery treats, and donuts and whole grains like oats, buckwheat, quinoa, and farro, which have genuine health benefits.

Clean Carbs

Your go-to source of carbs (and food in general) is produce. No matter your goals, your mindset, and your diet du jour, these superfoods should make their way onto your plate. Every. Single. Day. **All produce—fruits and vegetables—in its natural state is an ideal source of carbohydrates.** Apples, spinach, berries, kale, beets, and other garden gems available in the produce section at your local grocer offer varying amounts of energy along with fiber, antioxidants, phytochemicals, and nutrients to support your activity and your health. Occasionally produce comes under fire for having high calories (due to natural sugar in the form of fructose), or for causing weight gain—bananas and grapes are among the common targets. Case in point: I crossed paths with an influencer who promoted himself as a guru of nutrition—he had no formal training in the subject, but he did eat every day and his body composition was impressive . . . so I guess that makes him an expert on food. We were discussing different approaches to health and weight loss, and he told me that he warns all his personal training clients to avoid fruit because it's fruit that makes you fat. Yup. That happened. We are suffering from chronic disease and obesity because our intake of fruit is so damn high. You can stop worrying right now.

According to research from the Centers for Disease Control and Prevention, just 1 in 10 adults in the US meets the federal fruit and vegetable daily recommendations: 1½ to 2 cups of fruit and 2 to 3 cups of vegetables per day. In general, a serving of vegetables provides 5 grams of carbs and amounts to 1 cup of cooked or 2 cups of raw leafy greens. A serving of fruit typically contains 15 to 30 grams of carbs depending on the type and size of the fruit. A single serving is equal to 1 cup of chopped or sliced fresh fruit, 8 ounces of 100 percent fruit juice, ½ cup dried fruit, or one medium-size piece of whole fruit. Whether fresh, frozen, or canned, just about all produce is a clean carb.

High-Fiber Carbs

In addition to looking for better sources of carbohydrates, don't neglect to get fiber in your diet. You can find fiber in beans, nuts, seeds, fruits, veggies, and whole grains. Ideally, you should be eating at least 14 grams

How to get clean carbs

Choose whole foods. Fruit, veggies, and bulk grains will put you on the right path.

Check the label. Opt for foods with a short list of ingredients. Look for words like "whole-grain" rather than "enriched," which means the grain has been processed and stripped of naturally occurring nutrients, which are then replaced.

Skip foods with added sugar. Most of us should be consuming no more than 25 grams of added sugar a day.

Shop the perimeter of your grocery store. Many foods that are made to live on a grocer's shelf for months at a time are more likely to contain additives, refined grains, and added sugar.

Do a gut check. When you pick up a processed food or a sweet treat, ask yourself, Is this the best choice for me?

of fiber for every 1,000 calories you consume. For most of us, that equates to a goal of 25 to 30 grams of fiber per day. The vast majority (around 90 percent) of Americans do not come close to hitting this target. **Higher fiber intake is linked to lower body weight, so by simply meeting the goal of 30 grams a day, you might weigh 5 pounds less in a year's time.**

The fiber found in clean carbs works its weight-loss magic in multiple ways. Behind the scenes, high-fiber diets can lead to improved blood lipid levels. Physically, fiber helps you feel fuller for longer given that it takes more time to digest. Fiber-rich foods don't cause extreme spikes in blood sugar and consequent rises in the fat-depositing hormone insulin, which means that more fiber can lead to less intake and less fat storage. Winning!

Protein

Whether you fit the bill of athlete or fitness enthusiast, or you find yourself searching for changes that nurture transformation, you're going to need more protein to fuel your fitness. And due to bioavailability and how protein is absorbed in the body, you'll want to include diverse, high-quality sources and pace your intake throughout your day.

Protein is the nutrient du jour and for good reason; it is responsible for a plethora of metabolic reactions in addition to being essential for maintaining a strong immune system, bones, tendons, musculature, and the list goes on. There's also a clear link between adequate protein and satiety, lean body mass preservation, and weight loss. For this reason alone, you've likely seen an array of new sources of protein and plenty of new options professing to be high in protein. If you're highly active, the role protein plays is even more important. Workouts lead to exercise-induced muscle breakdown and demand rebuilding; small amounts of protein are used for energy, and additional protein beyond the bare minimum RDA is needed to support gains in lean muscle mass.

➡ How Much Do You Need?

When considering protein recommendations for the general population (i.e., somewhat sedentary) in comparison with the needs of a fitness enthusiast or an athlete in heavy training, activity easily trumps sitting on the couch. Research has equipped experts with the confidence to recommend an intake for athletes that handily doubles the needs of the general population. And an increased intake for those who are cutting calories and carbohydrates is similar. For athletes, increased protein accommodates adaption to workout load, repair and recovery of muscle, as well as a host of other performance-related changes. For those looking to lose weight, additional protein accounts for amino acids being metabolized for fuel and to enhance glycogen stores (via a process called gluconeogenesis) when overall carb intake is low.

You may have heard that most people, and especially athletes, eat too much protein. But the baseline for that judgment is typically the RDA for the general population, which is set at 0.36 grams per pound of body weight per day (0.8 g/kg/day). If you're consistently breaking a sweat or if you're middle age or older, your protein needs extend well beyond this baseline in order to support tissues with rapid turnover and augment metabolic adaptations initiated by training. Active individuals need to aim for an intake between 0.55 to 0.9 grams per pound per day (1.2–2.0 g/kg/day). Don't worry if you slightly surpass this upper threshold; more progressive nutrition experts have been recommending intakes of 1 gram per pound of lean body mass (and then some!) for years with great success. This level of protein intake assures that you have adequate amino acid levels to activate protein synthesis should energy or carb intake be so low that protein is oxidized as an energy source. An added bonus: Higher protein intake during periods of energy restriction or even during times of injury and those miserable off days may also help prevent losses in fat-free mass.

➤➤ What to Look For

With a plethora of new sources and marketing claims, how can you tell which proteins will give you the most health and performance benefits? After all, *quality* is not the same as *quantity*, and one gram of protein is not necessarily the same as another gram. Start with amino acid content. Amino acids are the building blocks of protein. When you eat a source of protein, your body breaks it down into individual amino acids, and these amino acids are stored in a pool in the body and used to reassemble new proteins and perform different functions. Sources of protein contain different amino acid combinations, and this combination determines if a protein is high quality. Nutrition expert and strength athlete Steve Hertzler, PhD, RD, explains that when considering protein sources, it's best to select those that are high enough in the essential amino acids to meet human requirements for growth and development. Adults do *grow* every day—whether it's renewing tissue or growing muscles after hours spent at the gym. We further *develop* our system as we progress toward our goals—whether that's improvements in fitness or VO_2max!

When looking for good sources of protein, first consider quality, which is a function of protein digestibility (highly digestible proteins contain amino acids readily available to the body), amino acid content, and the resulting amino acid availability to support metabolic function. But how do you know which sources of protein are high quality if you haven't spent decades immersed in nutrition research like Dr. Hertzler? It's easier than you might think. In general, animal sources are high in all the essential amino acids, while plant sources are commonly low in select essential amino acids, such as leucine—the amino acid that plays a critical role in turning on muscle protein synthesis. Additionally, plant proteins are more difficult to digest, so their bioavailability is also compromised. In other words, most animal sources are effective on their own, while plant protein sources often need to be combined with a different (plant) source of protein that contains alternate amino acids in order to deliver the benefits of a complete protein. Let's look at some protein sources so you can determine if your favorites are high quality or need work.

Animal Proteins

Animal proteins range from your typical beef, pork, chicken, eggs, and fish to drinkable dairy, bone broths, and shakes (typically whey and casein protein powders). And while plant protein sources continue to grow in popularity, animal sources—meat, fish, dairy, eggs—are still viewed by most consumers as top choices for protein. In fact, the trend of high-protein diets across the United States is driving some of the fastest rates of growth the meat industry has experienced in more than 40 years. Jerky alone is a $500 million market and growing. Meat sales are expected to surpass 200 pounds a year per capita.

Most of these animal sources, save for collagen and related bone broths, are high-quality protein sources that are well founded and highly bioavailable. Collagen protein, while popular and used for various reasons like joint health, is high in just three amino acids—glycine, proline, and hydroxyproline—while other animal proteins offer a more robust amino acid profile that better supports health and per-formance gains.

When it comes to protein from dairy, you really can't go wrong. It's high in essential amino acids—especially leucine—it's convenient and relatively inexpensive, and it has been extensively studied across multi-ple populations. Case in point, studies involving chronic exercisers have found that consumption of milk-based protein following resistance exercise is effective both in promoting muscle protein synthesis and in leading to improvements in body composition. These benefits hinge on the presence of casein and whey—two ingredients naturally present in milk. Casein, a slow-digesting protein, provides a steady stream of

Protein content
of different foods

So now that you're convinced you need more protein, let's do a calculation. Multiply your weight by the recommended range to determine your daily protein needs (g/d).

your weight in lb. × 0.55   MODERATE–
× 0.9   HIGH

your weight in kg × 1.2   MODERATE–
× 2.0   HIGH

Regardless of how your macronutrient goals sort out, try for at least one serving of protein per meal.

Poultry	26–27 g	3 oz. chicken breast (about half of breast) 4 oz. Cornish game hen
Meats	20–25 g	3.5–4 oz. steak (eye of round, filet) 3 oz. lean hamburger
Seafood	17–23 g	3 oz. canned tuna, drained 3 oz. salmon steak 3 oz. shrimp
Soy protein	17–21 g	¼ cup roasted soybeans ½ cup (4 oz.) tofu
Eggs	6–7 g	1 egg or 2 egg whites
Other plant protein	4–8 g	½ cup cooked beans (black, kidney, pinto, or white beans) ½ cup cooked peas (chickpeas, lentils, or split peas) ½ cup baked beans or refried beans 4 Tbsp. hummus
Nuts & seeds	4–7 g	1 oz. nuts (23 almonds, 49 pistachios, 14 walnut halves) 1 oz. seeds (83 pumpkin, sunflower, or squash seeds) 2 Tbsp. peanut butter or almond butter

Note: All values (according to the USDA FoodData Central) are for cooked or canned items unless otherwise indicated.

amino acids to muscles over many hours, while whey is known to be rapidly digested and therefore quickly repairs, restores, and rebuilds muscles after a workout.

Plant Proteins

Thanks to consumers who are seeking out more protein and looking to get it from varied sources, plant proteins are growing in popularity. But it's important to note that **plant-based protein is less anabolic than animal-based protein—in other words, plant protein is not as conducive to rebuilding and growth compared to animal proteins.** And that fact remains, even when it contains all of the essential amino acids, which is the case with soy. Soy protein is widespread in many sports nutrition supplements as well as in soy milk, tempeh, edamame, and more.

Excluding soy, plant-based proteins contain far fewer essential amino acids compared to animal-based protein. You could compensate by simply eating more, but without adequate variety, it won't matter how much of one specific source you consume—you'll still be missing essential amino acids. At the end of the day, most researchers, athletes, and especially vegan athletes agree that protein recommendations should not be seen as a fixed number. The amount of protein you need is dependent on the quality of protein in your diet. If you consume only plant-based protein, you'll need to eat more total daily protein to compensate for the lower protein quality and ensure adequate intake of amino acids. With careful planning and an openness to variety and new foods, this can be done! However, if you seek optimal protein intake but prefer to not worry about your mix of amino acids and overall protein quality, your best bet is to consume a variety of proteins throughout the day. Choose from an array of animal proteins containing essential amino acids as well as plant proteins offering select amino acids and, perhaps more important, additional health benefits.

Fat

Not too long ago, fats were considered a four-letter word. This energy-dense macronutrient, weighing in at 9 calories a gram, intimidated weight-loss warriors and athletes, who bought into the popular belief that eating fat would in fact made you fat. Talk about a shift in perspective: Today's dieters have sent the price of salmon, olive oil, and avocados soaring with their demand for healthy fats!

Tasty and nourishing fats should have a presence in your diet, whatever your specific health or wellness goal may be. Dietary fat plays many roles in the body, the first being as an energy source to help meet daily demands. This fat intake also has the ability to provide energy when your cells can't access other fuel sources, such as glucose, due to dietary restriction or illness or because of specific disease states. Fat stores help to maintain a consistent body temperature, and like it or not, our padding is perfectly designed to offer protection for internal organs.

Dietary fat intake and fat stores also allow for improved absorption of essential fat-soluble vitamins—the nutrients that are indispensable to optimal health, wellness, and even performance. Fat-soluble vitamin A is critical for vision as well as reproduction, cell differentiation, and bone formation. The hormone and sunshine vitamin, vitamin D, maintains bone health and calcium status yet is not widely available in most foods, so we want to be certain we absorb as much as possible. Dietary fat both supplies and helps with the absorption of antioxidant vitamin E, an immune-boosting nutrient. In fact, exercise may further increase your need for vitamin E. Last but not least, vitamin K should not be overlooked as it's necessary for blood clotting and bone health. Research has found that vitamin K supplementation and enhanced absorption is even more important in athletic populations since the metabolic cost of intense exercise can be draining on bone structure.

The type of fat you consume makes a difference. While unsaturated fats can improve your cholesterol and heart health, *trans* fats can raise the levels of total cholesterol. *Trans* fats are poor choices because they alter your total cholesterol ratio, decreasing the levels of healthy cholesterol (HDL) while increasing the levels of bad cholesterol (LDL) and ultimately increasing your risk of developing heart disease. We have yet to understand the full impact of saturated fats, but these solid fats have been shown to impact total cholesterol levels and may have the potential to negatively impact heart health. So it makes sense that we are cautioned to totally eliminate *trans* fats and to restrict saturated fat intake to no more than 10 percent of daily calories. The best fats and oils come from plants, not animals. **Dietary fats from plants, nuts, and seeds support optimal health because they largely are made up of unsaturated fats.** This means we aim to eat less bacon and butter and more avocados, olive oil, grapeseed oil, nut butters, and, on occasion, coconut oil.

➤➤ How Much Do You Need?

While the ketogenic high-fat diet calls for the vast majority of calories to come from fat, **the AMDR suggests that fat provide between 20 and 35 percent of your daily calories.** Failing to consume the minimum recommended intake can lead to undesirable outcomes. While low-fat diets have long been promoted for weight loss (due to the fact that a gram of fat is more energy dense than carbs or protein), this approach can lead to inadequate intake of micronutrients and essential fatty acids, which can increase your risk for injury. A 2008 study found that female runners who consumed a diet that was significantly lower in total fat and in percentage of total energy were 2.5 times more likely to be sidelined by injury as compared to runners who consumed 30 percent of their daily energy from fat. Ultimately, there is no performance benefit to a low-fat diet (which is defined as less than 15 percent of total energy intake). The best times to decrease your fat intake are pre-workout and pre-race meals, where the focus is on carbs, protein, and fluid, or right before a sweat session if you find that higher fat intake wreaks havoc on your GI system.

➤➤ **What to Look For**

Fats are sometimes grouped into "good" or "bad," pro-inflammatory or anti-inflammatory. While I find these labels to be problematic, it's safe to say that some fat choices should be "never foods" (*trans* fats), some should be "sometimes foods" (saturated and animal-based fats), and others get the green light as "always foods" (plant oils, fish oils, and unsaturated choices). Heart-healthy, nourishing, and nutrient-rich fats from nuts and oils can aid you in your quest to get lean and toned. Optimally, these fats should come from nutrient-dense food sources that supply vitamins and minerals along with macronutrients and energy.

Unsaturated Fats

In general, unsaturated fats are good choices, thanks to their positive impact on total cholesterol and LDL levels and their role in guarding against heart disease. You'll find unsaturated fats in vegetable and nut oils, such as almond, avocado, canola, olive, peanut, pecan, and pistachio. The umbrella term *unsaturated fat* includes both mono-unsaturated and polyunsaturated, classifications based on the chemical structure of these lipids. Most fats and oils contain a mix of both monounsaturated fatty acids (MUFA) and polyunsaturated fatty acids (PUFA), and since both types offer health benefits, there's no need to lose sleep trying to determine your exact intake of each.

The family of PUFA contains the essential fatty acids omega-3 and omega-6, which are particularly important because your body isn't able to make them. These fats regulate cellular functions and maintain brain, muscle, and nerve function. Eating more foods rich in these fatty acids, and omega-3, in particular, can lead to reduced risk of heart disease and protect against chronic inflammatory diseases and age-related brain decline. Sources of omega-6 oils are easy to find—plant oils like soy and canola—but you'll need to work a bit harder to find sources of omega-3 oils, which are found in fish oils and fatty cold-water fish, shellfish, walnuts, and flaxseed.

Trans Fat

When it comes to overly processed *trans* fat, you'll want to avoid it altogether as intake has been linked to poor blood lipid levels, increased risk of cardiovascular disease and stroke, and other undesirable outcomes. Look for foods with 0 grams per serving, but be aware that rounding comes into play. Foods with less than 0.5 grams per serving can still be labeled as *trans*-fat free. Eat enough of these sources throughout the day and you will have unintentionally consumed a significant amount. Higher levels of *trans* fat are typically only found in commercial baked goods, snack items, and margarines, all foods you're limiting anyway, right? While *trans* fats are naturally occurring in foods from ruminant animals (milk, butter, cheese, beef, etc.), it's the foods containing partially hydrogenated oils that you'll want to watch out for.

Medium-Chain Fatty Acids

These oils are typically relied upon for quick supply of energy as well as for their potential to improve metabolic burn. Medium-chain trigycerides (MCTs) can be found in select household oils (coconut and palm kernel oil as well as, to some extent, butter) and also in powdered and liquid supplements. The benefit of a diet rich in MCT oil revolves around the oil's chemical structure—MCTs are chemically smaller lipids compared to other saturated and unsaturated fats. Due to their shorter chain length, MCTs can be absorbed in the gastrointestinal tract and transported to the liver via the portal circulation without extra steps typically required to digest a longer chain source of fat. As a result, MCTs are quickly used for energy by the muscles, surrounding tissues, and even the brain (while in a ketogenic state), rather than being stored and then contributing to padding!

Recent research suggests that there may be metabolic advantages to switching from an intake of typical longer-chain oils to MCT oil. In a small trial where 31 individuals consumed 18 to 24 grams per day of either olive oil or MCT oil, those who consumed MCT oil maintained a lower body weight and were on trend to improve body composition as well. Other research points to the ability of MCT oil to fight fat storage, increase thermogenesis (metabolic burn), and increase satiety. In fact, a clinical trial found that including a daily dose of MCT oil may result in negative energy balance and weight loss through increased energy expenditure and lipid oxidation. And frequent replacement of dietary fat with sources of MCTs could potentially induce modest reductions in body weight and composition without adversely affecting lipid profile. There's no harm to including more variety in your diet. If you're looking for a place to start, many people consume MCT oil in the morning for a quick shot of energy as well as focus. Powdered or liquid, MCT oil mixes well into hot beverages and is commonly found in high-fat butter-coffee. But not everyone's GI tract tolerates MCT oil well. For best results, start by slowly incorporating this fat into your diet, and over time any GI distress you might experience is sure to improve.

Saturated Fat

It's easy to spot saturated fats because they are typically solid at room temperature. Sources include butter, lard, bacon, fatty cuts of meat, poultry with the skin, dairy products, as well as coconut oil, palm oil, and cocoa butter. (Coconut oil is a versatile fat that is rich in medium-chain triglycerides but also higher in saturated fat.) **The *Dietary Guidelines for Americans 2015–2020*, 8th edition, recommends that your diet include less than 10 percent of daily calories from saturated fat.** This means that for every 1,000 calories you consume, your intake should be less than 11 grams. This is the amount found in 1½ tablespoons of butter, 1 tablespoon of coconut oil, or ⅓ cup of heavy cream.

In the past, restrictions on saturated fat intake were severe, with health and nutrition experts urging people to avoid these foods as much as possible. It was recommended that these foods be replaced with unsaturated fats and even shelf-stable *trans* fats found in foods like margarine. But this advice has come under fire.

A recent meta-analysis published in the *Annals of Internal Medicine* found that people who ate higher levels of saturated fat did not have more heart disease than those who ate less. Nor did it find less disease in those eating higher amounts of unsaturated fat, including monounsaturated fats, such as avocados and olive oil, or polyunsaturated fats, such as soybean and canola oils. If you think this means you get the green light to load up on all the bacon and lard you can stomach, think again. Decades of research still support the stance that you'll lower your risk of heart disease by replacing saturated fats with heart-healthy fats in nuts, seeds, avocados, fish, plant oils, and vegetable-oil soft spreads. Still, this meta-analysis is part of a growing body of research that has challenged the oft-repeated advice that saturated fat should be virtually eliminated. Nutrition and communications expert Jenna Bell, PhD, RD, notes, "Years of research on fat in the diet have shown that increasing 'good fats' (like those found in nuts, seeds, avocados, fish, and plant oils) is a heart-healthy choice." She adds that even with the emergence of science inquiries taking a closer look at the value of high-fat dairy and the popularity of coconut oils, few studies have shown that saturated fat is necessary for health. While the scientists duke it out, endorsing a diet high in saturated fat remains unwarranted. "Think about variety and diversity when grocery shopping, doing meal prep, and eating out—not just single nutrients. Aim for an interesting approach to food and look for protein from a variety of sources—including plant-based options like nuts (nut butters, nut milks, handfuls) and pulses (beans, legumes, lentils, and dried peas) along with meats and dairy options (if you choose). Avoid getting stuck in a rut or only choosing foods based on one nutrient only," says Dr. Bell. In other words, if you are currently following a diet loaded with saturated fat, the evidence and experts recommend emphasizing plant-based options or seafood for fat. The bottom line, according to Dr. Bell: "It's not about one nutrient—we need to focus on all the foods in our diet and aim for a delicious variety of healthful foods."

Be open. Be purposeful.
And find <u>your own</u> best macro mix.

The Macro Mix for Endurance & Performance

Do the numbers 13.1, 26.2, 70.3 (or more) stoke more happy thoughts than angst for you? Are you determined to hit a PR in the season ahead? If you are deep in training or focused on a performance goal, start your search for the optimal macro mix right here.

Long-course endurance events, relays, and obstacle course challenges are neither for the faint of heart nor for the unprepared. To line up for such a challenge means committing to months of training, logging hundreds of miles, and downing thousands of ounces of fluid, hundreds of grams of carbohydrates, countless grams of protein, and enough calories to support the effort.

The precise amount of fluid and energy needed to carry you through weeks of training and hours of sweat sessions is a science. Tweaks must be made to individualize recommendations, and these needs evolve over time. The beauty of using a food journal while training for an event is the ability to track your intake before, during, and after a session and record what works and what didn't. Maybe you ate too little before a long run and totally bonked halfway in. By writing it down and referencing it later, you'll realize the next time out that you need a bit more pre-run grub. Or maybe you tried a certain brand of gel during a long hike and found yourself scurrying for the bushes! You'll know to avoid it the next time adventure calls.

What follows is a detailed look at the recommended ranges of macronutrients and fluids needed to support intense and consistent training. Follow these guidelines and you'll arrive at your next challenge ready to conquer the day.

Carbohydrates

It's easy to get overwhelmed by the myriad choices available to fuel a long run, ride, or any other activity lasting longer than 90 minutes. Bars, gels, drinks, and chews exist to provide quick, easy-to-digest energy. This energy stems from carbohydrates, the primary fuel used during physical activity, and adequate amounts are needed for optimal performance. Carbohydrates are stored in muscles and the liver in the form of glycogen, and the amount that can be stored varies, dependent upon overall fitness, intensity of training, and dietary intake. Because these stores are limited, carbohydrates must be consumed daily as well as before, during, and after longer training runs and races. The following ranges of carb intake are for athletes of all shapes and sizes.

 RECOMMENDED CARBOHYDRATE INTAKE

Most endurance athletes logging an hour or more of exercise per day need 5 to 10 grams of carbs per kilogram of body weight per day (g/kg/day), which equates to about 2.3 to 4.5 grams per pound per day (g/lb./day). Invest in yourself and your performance by sitting down with a sports dietitian to further personalize this range, based on your response to macronutrient distribution, body composition goals, training level, and the type of event.

FUEL	Moderate training, 1 hr.	Moderate to high-intensity training, 1–3 hr.
	CARBS 5–7 g/kg/day	CARBS 7–10 g/kg/day

Protein

Whether you consider yourself a fitness enthusiast or a marathon junkie, protein intake is critical. This essential nutrient is responsible for muscle rebuilding and repair, and during times of heavy training, an increase in protein is certainly warranted. Plus, if you've decided to reduce your carbs but you still want to train long or intensely, you'll need to bump up your protein in order to maintain lean muscle mass and protect your glycogen levels.

➡ RECOMMENDED PROTEIN INTAKE

The general population can get by with a bare minimum of 0.8 grams per kilogram per day (0.36 g/lb./day), but if you've got a big training load, you need more. Much more. Aim for at least 1.2 to 2.0 grams per kilogram per day (0.55–0.91 g/lb./day) and focus on the higher end of this range during periods of intense training or when reducing overall energy intake. Include protein at each meal, supplement with a protein shake here and there, track your intake, and you should have little difficulty coming close to these recommended protein intakes. If you're a vegetarian or vegan athlete, switch up your sources of protein throughout the day and track your grams so you know when you hit your goal.

Fat

A necessary source of fuel, fat, along with carbohydrates, is oxidized during exercise to provide energy to working muscles. Over the long haul (i.e., workouts and races lasting longer than 90 minutes), carbohydrate stores are often quickly depleted, and the body turns to fat for fuel. At 9 calories per gram, fat packs quite a punch in terms of caloric density and energy provision.

⇒ RECOMMENDED FAT INTAKE

Fat-containing foods are vital to all diets as they provide energy and aid in the absorption of key nutrients such as vitamins A, D, E, and K. Consistent research has not yet found compelling performance benefits when athletes follow a ketogenic diet (greater than 70 percent of total calories from fat) and certainly not when following a very low-fat diet (less than 15 percent of total energy intake). Instead, aim for moderation. Start with an intake consistent with the Acceptable Macronutrient Distribution Range (AMDR) for fat: 20 to 35 percent of total calories. The best way to accomplish this is to get fat from heart-healthy, anti-inflammatory sources, such as plant oils, avocados, and nuts, and to limit excessive intake of saturated fat, *trans* fat, and animal fats.

Micronutrients

It is well known that vitamins and minerals play critical roles in energy production, growth, and development, as well as maintenance and protection of bones, tissues, organs, blood, and the immune system. Long-course racing and the training it demands can increase the need for these nutrients due to losses in urine and sweat as well as the cost to repair tissue. Most of the time, if you consume enough (well-balanced) calories to fuel your sport, the respective RDA or dietary reference intake (DRI) will suffice. But if you're cutting calories, following a restrictive diet, or just don't have a good handle on what balanced eating looks like, then you'll likely want to consider supplementation.

DV Versus DRI—What's the Difference?

Dietary Reference Intake (DRI) establishes the guidelines for how much of each nutrient you need, while the Daily Value (DV)—often listed as a percentage on a food label—tells you how much of the nutrients you're actually getting from the foods you eat.

RECOMMENDED MICRONUTRIENT INTAKE

Common micronutrients that need to be closely monitored and possibly supplemented include calcium, iron, vitamin D, and various antioxidants. Deficiencies are most common in female athletes, athletes severely reducing their overall energy intake, and athletes following restrictive diets. These shortages can have dire consequences, like stress fractures or hormone disruption. A low intake of total calories and especially animal products, including red meat and dairy, is often at fault. By consuming a diet rich in a variety of foods (especially whole grains and complete proteins) micronutrient deficiencies can typically be avoided.

Fluid

If you've ever attempted to PR or perform while suffering the ill effects of dehydration (headache, fatigue, poor performance) you probably promised yourself "never again." Avoid the slower race times, decreased muscle strength, decreased stamina, and decreased cognitive function that accompany improper hydration. It doesn't take much fluid loss to spell out impaired performance—just 1 to 2 percent of body weight lost from fluid can mess with your mental strength, heart rate, and overall performance, especially in hot weather. But not to worry: Research shows that by preventing and replacing sweat losses with proper fluid and electrolyte intake, all of these issues and complications can be alleviated.

RECOMMENDED FLUID INTAKE

Most of us lose somewhere between 0.3 to 2.4 liters (10 to 81 ounces) of fluid per hour during exercise, depending on factors such as intensity, duration, heat acclimatization, altitude, weather conditions, and various physiological parameters. Ideally, you'll want to drink to meet your thirst cues and keep sweat loss to less than 2 percent. In order to know how much sweat you're losing and how much to replace, perform the DIY Sweat Test on p. 101. Once you've got your number in hand, don't just chug copious amounts of water with the goal of preventing dehydration. Overhydration can dilute plasma sodium stores and result in a serious condition known as hyponatremia. Instead, add electrolytes—sodium, chloride, and potassium at a minimum— to your water. Pedialyte is a great choice as it's absorbed quickly from the gut (no sloshing!). You can also shop around: look for a supplement that contains high levels of sodium and chloride, moderate levels of potassium, and a hint of other nutrients, if included.

The average athlete shows up to the workout <u>dehydrated</u>. Don't be average.

The DIY sweat test

It's best to perform a sweat test under conditions that mimic the environment in which you'll be competing. Since you can't be certain of future weather conditions, plan to repeat this test throughout training in order to more precisely determine the fluid you'll need on race day. The goal is to maintain your hydration status, avoiding both overhydration (which increases the potential for dangerous hyponatremia) and dehydration (which is sure to derail performance or land you with a DNF).

1

Warm up, hydrate, and urinate as normal before a one-hour workout. Weigh yourself naked on your scale.

2

Perform a one-hour workout at race-day intensity. Don't urinate or eat solids during the session, but consume fluids as normal. Pay careful attention to the amount of fluid you consume.

3

At the end of the workout, weigh yourself naked again, using the same scale.

4

Calculate your post-workout weight loss; then add in the fluid ounces consumed during activity.

5

If the total number is lower than your starting weight, increase your fluid intake by the amount of the deficit. For longer events, keep in mind that you will need to cover the amount of fluid lost for each hour of activity.

Sample Sweat Test

Starting weight: 140 lb.

Intake during hour-long run: 12 oz.

Ending weight: 139 lb.

Sweat losses:
1 lb. (16 oz.) + 12 oz. (0.75 lb.) = loss of 28 oz.

Intake recommendation =
28 oz. per hour to maintain hydration

There are 16 ounces in a pound and 8 ounces in a cup.

X Factors to Make (or Break) Your Goals

Most of us know the type of foods we should be consuming. We may even have a good idea of the nutrients we need. And the amounts. Even the portions. And we may put into practice good habits to avoid mindless noshing. If only health, performance, and reaching a feel-good weight were as simple as having the know-how.

In reality, our ability to eat healthy and remain active day in and day out is affected by other facets of our lifestyle. Get everything right and these three things wrong and you could easily fall back into mindless eating, plate envy, or choosing the couch over the gym. So if you want to move confidently toward your goals, you have to better manage your support, sleep, and stress. All the time and energy you put into working out and eating well will be leveraged by these three X factors.

Support

Let me be completely honest with you: **Support makes the journey infinitely more enjoyable.** You're going to need someone to pat you on the back, tell you to stay the course, and exclaim that your calves look amazing in those shoes! When you decide to embark upon on a new habit of eating or otherwise choose to create healthier habits, it's crucial that you get some buy-in from those who matter to you—be it your partner in crime, your family, your coworkers, or whomever. But how to get everyone on board? And how do you follow your own way of eating but balance the requests of others in your household?

Share Your Goal

Begin by explaining your *why*. Your reason for seeking something better. Dig deep for this one, make your why compelling and passionate and rock-solid, and then have a sit-down conversation. These changes are not selfishly motivated; they are for everyone's benefit. Remind yourself and others in the room that as you sail toward better, the wake you leave behind makes for smoother sailing for everyone on board. By improving yourself, you improve your attitude, your interactions, and your impact on others' health and performance. You become a model of what's possible with better health.

People Are Aid Stations

At this face-to-face, map out the changes you'd like to make and even the intricacies of your approach. Stop being a one-person show and a martyr and instead be upfront about the help you'll need and why support is critical. As evidence of this, a study among women undergoing a 12-week weight loss program found that 74 percent of them maintained their weight loss or went on to lose more in the three years after the program ended thanks to having a support system around eating well.

Articulate what it is you need for support. Do you need your partner to handle morning mayhem while you train for your first-ever race and log predawn miles? Discuss the help you'll provide in return. Maybe you've identified that you simply cannot have certain trigger foods in the house. You'll need buy-in from others in your household. After all, until you've confidently cemented a new habit, you need time to build the strength needed to say no to old favorites. Together, identify better choices, the middle ground that will work for everyone.

Take a Test Run

Ease everyone into your new way of eating by making a meal that fully meets your needs yet incorporates what they are familiar with too. For example, if you are going keto, not everyone needs to go full fat. In fact, some lifestyles are not designed to support the needs of everyone in your household. No matter the nutritional lifestyle you choose to follow, there's a strong likelihood that something on the menu will speak to everyone. In the case of keto, it's likely bacon, avocado, or sirloin steak. And there's really no harm in cutting out simple sugars and meals consisting solely of refined grains and empty calories. To help with the transition, include a side dish that they enjoy. This thoughtful act will let your tribe see that even though you are eating differently, you can continue to eat together without anyone feeling ostracized.

Lean into Your Why

You're striving to create a new outlook and a new outcome, and at times that will feel like a lonely road. You might have friends who whine about how you no longer binge-drink or bury your sorrows in sweet indulgences. Don't let these vibes bring you down. Change the tone or distance yourself where possible.

Patiently continue to share your goals and invite others along. Some will join; others will choose to carry on with their lives as usual. Accept that and move on. Channel your energy into being stronger than those who attempt to drag you back into old habits. There's a reason you want to leave the old you behind—let it drive you forward.

Sleep

Chasing better fitness or a better diet or better health is fruitless if you don't incorporate better sleep habits as well. Swapping sleep for time in the gym, in the kitchen, or practicing wellness is like trying to get rich by stepping over $100 bills to pick up all the pennies. It's a futile pursuit. So why do 9 in 10 Americans prioritize just about any other aspect of daily living (fitness/nutrition, work, social life, and hobbies/personal interests) over precious sleep?! Experts, such as those at the National Sleep Foundation, which uncovered this alarming finding, know that the value of sleep can't be overstated. Of course, fewer waking hours allow for less access to food, but it's so much more than that. **Reduced sleep can amp up cravings and hunger and rob you of the energy needed to work out.**

Research studying the association between self-reported typical sleep duration and subsequent weight gain found that over time, a chronically shorter night's sleep can lead to weight gain. The data, from the Nurses' Health Study, included more than 68,000 RNs and a span of 16 years. The subjects who reported sleeping less gained more weight than those who reported sleeping more. In fact, getting even one additional hour of sleep per night made a significant impact: Over the course of the study, women who slept five hours or less a night gained 2.5 pounds more than did those who slept seven hours, while women who slept six hours a night gained 1.5 pounds more. Interestingly, these associations were not affected by amount of time spent working out or by diet, suggesting that shorter sleep durations alone (rather than the fact that you're too tired to work out or that you're chronically snacking) impact the rate of weight gain. Other studies have found similar results, going so far as to suggest that adults sleeping less than seven hours per night are more likely to be obese. However, in these studies, it could be a question of the chicken versus the egg—battling excess weight can lead to sleep apnea and arthritis, and these two conditions alone can make it difficult to sleep. While it's not certain which came first, lack of sleep or excess weight, what you need to know is that it's crucial that you get your z's.

Maybe your problem is that you can't sleep even if you make the time. If you're tracking your sleep and realize that you routinely come up short of seven or eight hours, it's time to get serious about your bedtime ritual. Here are four tried-and-true strategies for better sleep.

Prioritize

Just as you would set aside time for a workout or a tour of the health food store, set aside time for sleep. Make it habitual, starting your turndown ritual at the same time each day, and make it a goal to do this Monday through Sunday, especially if you've got a huge health or performance goal on your radar. More activity calls for more rest and recovery.

Tired? Make a plan

Shorter sleep duration can lead to decreased levels of leptin (a protein hormone that signals satiety) and increased levels of ghrelin (a gut peptide associated with the sensation of hunger). Not only will you be hungrier, but you'll also crave high-calorie, higher-carb choices, derailing those body comp goals you've been pursuing. There's no undoing last night's late night, but you can go into a tired day knowing that you're in danger of indulging. So take a few minutes to set a plan in place before too many late nights cause you to collapse into the office donuts.

Choose your drink wisely

Caffeine and alcohol can totally ruin a good night's sleep. Cut off caffeine before one or two in the afternoon, and the more sensitive you are to caffeine's effects the earlier you should shut it down. Grab a relaxing beverage like chamomile tea or casein-rich warm milk instead of alcohol if you need to be lulled to sleep. Alcohol may make you sleepy, but this dangerous habit produces short-lived effects with poor sleep quality and a lethargic and dehydrated morning to follow. Keep the quantity of any extracurricular beverages reasonable and be sure to use the bathroom before you tuck in for the night.

Shut down your devices

You already know that the blue light of the phone and tablet are distracting and that the content can be stressful. Avoid being irked and irritated right before bed, and if you like to unwind by reading something, choose something other than your social feed. Instead, grab a relaxing magazine or novel. And if you simply cannot shut down your system and relax, find yourself an old textbook. Just like in your college days, it's sure to put you to sleep in no time.

Stress

When it comes to the dynamic of food and stress, there's the rare individual who deals with stress by shutting down all intake and not stomaching anything, and there's the far more common individual who eats to deal with whatever hand they've been dealt. And if you seek out food as a coping mechanism, you can thank your physiology. **Stress naturally increases the levels of cortisol circulating in your body and simultaneously drives your will to eat.** Extended or excessive bouts of stress can lead to accumulation of fat tissue, increased hunger, periods of binge-eating, an inability to make good food choices, and sometimes total loss of control when faced with indulgences. But enough about me!

A large study of 457 individuals resulted in similar findings. The study, involving normal to overweight women between the ages of 20 and 56 years old, assessed the relationship between stress (perceived and chronic), drive to eat, and reported food frequency intake (nutritious food versus tasty but nonnutritious food) and found that greater levels of reported stress, whether legit or perceived, were associated with indices of greater drive to eat. This increased drive included feelings of disinhibited eating, binge-eating, hunger, and ineffective attempts to control eating. For those of us battling chronic stress—the feeling of being under the gun and run-down for months at a time—there's a high probability of seeing higher numbers on the scale if something doesn't change. But even acute stress can lead us toward a path riddled with excessive intake of poor choices. Research suggests that acute stress alters food preferences toward sugary and fatty foods, increases eating frequency, and impacts the number of calories we consume. This response to stress varies across individuals, and your personal go-to stress foods are likely to be completely different from someone else's. There will always be exceptions to the rule—research has found that some of us respond to stress by decreasing intake. Maybe you fall into that lucky minority.

You can't hide from the stress of life, but you can deal with it . . . or so I've been told. With work, a relationship with stress can be simplified to you versus your stressor alone, and with practice you'll grow strong enough to leave your food wingman behind! Where to begin? Instead of coping with calories, choose one of the healthy strategies that follow and measure your success with the Monthly Habit Tracker pages throughout the journal (pp. 134, 171, 208).

Sweat it out

Your most powerful ally in the fight against stress is exercise. Exercise has the power to reduce levels of cortisol as well as increase feel-good hormones. You know that runner's high or those happy vibes you get after a solid workout? The feeling is real. So instead of coping with calories, work out those problems over a few miles or a few reps.

Relax already!

Whether you seek out meditation, a calming series of deep breaths, or repose through yoga, relaxation techniques allow a moment to pause and perhaps find a fresh perspective to bring your stress back into balance.

Talk it out

Find a friend who's removed from whatever is ailing you and spill. Explain what you're going through and ask for help. Whether you need advice, intercession, or a shoulder to cry on, a human being makes a better listener than a bowl of ice cream or potato chips. And you aren't left with feelings of guilt and regret afterward.

Sleep it off

Everything seems more clear and bright in the morning, doesn't it? That's because sleep affords you time to relax, reduce your levels of stress hormones, lower your body temperature, and start anew. Sleep provides a calorie-free way to reflect, relax, and map out a plan for tackling the issue with a clear mind.

Lay down the miles today to prepare for a <u>better tomorrow</u>.

Feed Your Hunger, Not Your Feelings

If only eating were as simple as listening to hunger cues and then consuming foods to satisfy your body's fundamental needs. Imagine! A world where nutrition books would cover macro- and micronutrients, detail the digestive system, and then lay out the recommended intakes to promote health. That's it. There would be no discussion on emotional eating, mindless grazing, the avoidance of trigger foods. There would be fewer chronic diseases, and the incidence of obesity wouldn't be the epidemic it is today. But alas, the art of eating is not as simple as balancing nutrient-dense calories in with metabolic cost of calories out. Instead, we live in a world where the line between hunger and appetite gets blurred, and coping with whatever the day hands us manifests as the need to soothe ourselves with food. Hence, emotional eating.

Think about the last time you craved chocolate while lonely, snacked instead of tackling your to-do list, or numbed a stressful day with comfort food—just like Mom used to make. If emotions play a huge role in your day-to-day decision making, these leading characters might be driving your calorie intake rather than simply coming along for the occasional ride. Many times, rather than eating due to hunger, we eat to numb our pain (or boredom, or anger, or happiness). We eat because we're starving for a break from what ails us—such as an awkward situation, an emotion that makes us squirm, or intense happiness. It's understandable that we seek an immediate solution to every discomfort—our society is designed to provide easy escapes (smartphone anyone?) rather than a way to deal with our emotions. And it's more socially acceptable to self-medicate with ice cream rather than life-derailing fifths of vodka or illicit drugs.

Another mind-boggling issue at hand is the fact that many of the foods we seek during times of stress contain some of the exact ingredients—sugars—that have been shown to light up the same areas of the brain as cocaine and other drugs and therefore result in similar withdrawal symptoms and cravings for more. And over time, the hypothesis goes, we become desensitized to the effects, therefore seeking more and more of the "good stuff" to increase the release of dopamine, the neurotransmitter known to play a role in boosting mood, given the role it plays in reward-motivated behavior. The problem is, emotional eating provides just a temporary feeling of pleasure, leaving you to deal with the real task at hand. These indulgences are simply distractions, and once the momentary pleasure you get from that sweet treat disappears, the stress, the to-do list, and the emotions are still there. And often, the original problem is compounded by the guilt you now have thanks to indulging in a sweet treat that wasn't in the meal plan.

Susan Albers, Cleveland Clinic psychologist and author of *Eating Mindfully* and five other books about emotional eating, counsels, "It can be very confusing to sort out the signals and determine—is it hunger or is it emotion?" Nutrition expert Lizzie Briasco, MSc, RD, adds that learning about and *practicing* mindfulness techniques can be very helpful. She notes that a solid starting point is distinguishing between physical and emotional hunger. If underfueling has been ruled out (i.e., you *have* had enough to meet your nutrient needs) and instead emotions have been identified as the driving force behind eating behaviors, identifying those feelings and emotional needs in that moment can make a huge difference! Lauren Vallee, an endurance athlete and coach with

BASE Tri Fitness, suggests using a hunger scale and an emotional scale and work to reconcile the two. Says Vallee, ask yourself, "How emotional am I on a scale of 1 to 10 (10 being full-on meltdown) and then how hungry am I on a scale of 1 to 10 (10 being I need to eat now or I will pass out)." If you're more emotional than hungry, meditate for five minutes, go for a walk, or make a cup of tea. If more hungry than emotional (but still triggered emotionally), pick a sensible (i.e., high-nutrient density, high-protein and fat, low-sugar) snack to keep energy steady.

Because mindless eating, emotional eating, and trigger foods can derail our day, our diet, and our goals, better outcomes arrive when we learn to thwart our eating instincts and instead grow to recognize true hunger instead. Luckily, the path has been laid before us by experts who have put in the work needed to identify food triggers and emotional triggers and stop them before they gain steam. Once you become aware of the emotional and environmental triggers setting up roadblocks between you and your goals and take a deep dive into what drives you and your disposition, you can use this information to create habits that set you up for success. Your goal is to create a series of curated habits, moving you toward your best and healthiest self. Follow the advice of board-certified sports dietitian Andrea Chapin: "As humans we will always favor routine and the path of least resistance; your healthy routine has to be the easiest one with the least amount of decisions. Healthy choices need to be on autopilot." Here's a list of expert-vetted strategies to follow to avoid, as Vallee puts it, a full-on emotional eating meltdown and instead move toward healthy eating on autopilot.

Every accomplishment starts with the _decision to try_.

Pro tips on winning the emotional game

Are you hungry or ... ? Consider your grumbling stomach, your energy level, your "hangry-ness," and compare it to your stressors, your emotions. By keeping track, you may discover a pattern driving your choices.

Set a timer. Nutrition and communications expert Rachel Bassler, MS, RD, suggests taking a walk, doing some yoga, or grabbing a good book for 20 minutes. When the timer goes off, if you find yourself really hungry, then indulge without guilt. A 20-minute time gap forces you to remove yourself from the situation should the pull be emotional rather than a true physical need.

Remember the celery rule. When we are truly hungry, just about anything sounds good; celery, carrots, string cheese. But if only something sweet or salty or [insert flavor here] will do, then you're experiencing a craving. Cravings are born out of habits and associations of the pleasure that said food will bring. So if it's hunger, grab some celery or some other healthy snack.

Don't eat your reward. This leads to bad habits: You'll likely eat more calories than you burned and negate your calorie deficit, and you'll set up a dangerous precedent of linking food with behavior. So link your hard work to something calorie-free and more permanent.

A new shirt after 10 strength sessions. Or a massage after a 20-miler. But skip the muffins after miles.

Maybe you're thirsty? The value of water goes far beyond basic hydration. It physically fills you, allowing you to then pause and ask, *Am I really hungry, or did I simply need to quench my thirst?* The signals for thirst and hunger are similar, allowing some of us to mistake an innate need for hydration with a need for food. Think about the last time you had a sweaty workout and forgot to rehydrate 110 percent. If you were overly "hungry" in the hours following said workout, it's likely that you needed fluid over foods.

Winning the emotional game *(continued)*

Kitchen's closed!
Once you've met your macros and answered the call of hunger, there's no need to keep eating. The foods we consume in the late hours of the day are typically more indulgent choices, emotionally or mindlessly driven—and worst of all, because we are not immediately using this energy, it's stored in the form of fat. So shut down the kitchen after dinner. Put up a sign. Lock the doors.

Change your environment.
A behavioral therapist once reported that a client sat on a couch every evening and overate, so they literally moved the couch out of the room. Reshaping your environment can change your behavior, counsels Andrea Chapin, RD. She reminds clients, "Think of how your environment sets you up for success or failure and make minor (or major!) adjustments that work for you."

Make mindful your mantra. Are you filling up out of habit or just because the clock says noon? Perusing the pantry shelves in a daze? Wolfing down without even tasting it? Shift back into the moment and reassess what else is going on.

Eat at the table!
Sanitation aside, eating at the table allows for a more mindful connection with food. We naturally associate eating in the context of our environment, and when no room, chair, nook, or cranny is immune to eating, you'll be triggered to eat. So do as your momma told you.

Give yourself a break. We are always our own harshest critic. Be kind to yourself. Journaling your food intake means that you are already rising to the challenge of becoming a better you.

THE ULTIMATE PRO TIP

Take baby steps. Research shows that successful weight loss comes when making a few purposeful changes and sticking with them for the long-term. At the beginning of each month, identify some small changes you can make each and every day. Positive changes build over time. Your mantra is *Progress, not perfection.*

What Kind of Eater Are You?

Deep down, maybe you know what type of eater you are. Maybe you realize that "stress eating" is forcing you to wear leggings 24/7 because you refuse to buy larger pants. Or maybe you are snacking while reading this, and you know it's the incremental mindless calories that are to blame. Or maybe you know that your less-than-healthy choices are the culprit. Then again, maybe you're scratching your head with no idea of what may be holding you back. Whatever your status, you're not alone.

Most of us have some idea of the types of foods we should choose more or less often. I call these "always foods" and "sometimes foods" to get away from the stigma of classifying foods into good and bad. It sounds simple, but making the right choice consistently without making it bigger than it needs to be is hard! Even if you have a PhD in nutrition, you can still run into setbacks. Simply knowing which foods belong on your plate and which nutrients you need, down to the milligram, will neither make you a healthy eater nor give you a great relationship with food. No matter who you are, mindless eating and emotional eating can derail your mind and body. If you know you're predisposed to eating this way, you can put practices in place to change these habits that hold you back.

Start by taking the following quiz, which is adapted from a questionnaire commonly used in research studies and is one I've crafted for use in my practice. It's useful in establishing a starting point to explore factors that might be holding you back from fully meeting your goals. It's here to help you better identify what might be going on behind the scenes and therefore driving what's on your plate. Be honest because the only one keeping score is you.

What kind of eater are you?

I eat so quickly I don't even taste my food!

A USUALLY/ALWAYS **B** OFTEN **C** SOMETIMES **D** NEVER/RARELY

Don't put the bowl of candy next to me or I will give in to the temptation!

A USUALLY/ALWAYS **B** OFTEN **C** SOMETIMES **D** NEVER/RARELY

I like to really taste and enjoy my food, savoring every bite.

A USUALLY/ALWAYS **B** OFTEN **C** SOMETIMES **D** NEVER/RARELY

All-you-can-eat buffets are trouble—once I start, I can't stop.

A USUALLY/ALWAYS **B** OFTEN **C** SOMETIMES **D** NEVER/RARELY

I tend to do a million things at once, including multitasking while eating.

A USUALLY/ALWAYS **B** OFTEN **C** SOMETIMES **D** NEVER/RARELY

I snack out of habit—even when I'm not hungry!

A USUALLY/ALWAYS **B** OFTEN **C** SOMETIMES **D** NEVER/RARELY

When I *finally* sit down to a meal and eat, the stress of my day either causes me to lose my appetite or drives me to eat more.

A USUALLY/ALWAYS **B** OFTEN **C** SOMETIMES **D** NEVER/RARELY

I have trouble saying no to sweet treats and other foods I crave if they are in the house.

A USUALLY/ALWAYS **B** OFTEN **C** SOMETIMES **D** NEVER/RARELY

When I'm eating foods I love, I often indulge too much, not realizing when I feel full.

A USUALLY/ALWAYS **B** OFTEN **C** SOMETIMES **D** NEVER/RARELY

If there's good food at a party, you can probably find me next to the buffet table!

A USUALLY/ALWAYS **B** OFTEN **C** SOMETIMES **D** NEVER/RARELY

When I'm bored or stressed or procrastinating, I go find something to eat.

A USUALLY/ALWAYS **B** OFTEN **C** SOMETIMES **D** NEVER/RARELY

They can't fool me! I know when
food ads inspire me to eat.

A	B	C	D
USUALLY/ ALWAYS	OFTEN	SOMETIMES	NEVER/ RARELY

Presentation matters. I love the
way good food looks on my plate
(and on Instagram!).

A	B	C	D
USUALLY/ ALWAYS	OFTEN	SOMETIMES	NEVER/ RARELY

Clean plate club be damned,
I stop eating when I'm satisfied.

A	B	C	D
USUALLY/ ALWAYS	OFTEN	SOMETIMES	NEVER/ RARELY

When I'm sad, eating my favorite
foods is a cure-all for the blues.

A	B	C	D
USUALLY/ ALWAYS	OFTEN	SOMETIMES	NEVER/ RARELY

SCORING METRIC

**Your score is not a diagnosis, nor is it meant to pile on shame.
Instead, consider it a thought starter and a prompt to set things right.**

MOSTLY A'S

It's all mood. I've been where
you are, and however far I've come,
I occasionally find myself right back
at the starting line. The fight against
mindless eating, stress eating,
emotional eating (or "whatever ails
you" kind of eating) can be a real
knockout boxing match. The good
news is that you don't have to deal
with all of the feels at once. Choose
a few of these emotional eating
habits and stress-eating habits
to address each week. Reassess
regularly, and when you pick off one
emotion or stressor, set your sights
on another. Use the nutrition goal-
setting section of the journal and the
Monthly Habit Tracker pages to get
started. Again, just a few small steps
at a time. You got this.

What kind of eater are you? *(continued)*

MOSTLY B'S

Struggling ever forward.

You're rocking some aspects of emotional and mindless eating. And you're likely more aware than you once were, but don't you agree there's more work to be done? Good thing you're up for the challenge! Use the daily habit tracker or the nutrition goal setting section of the journal and set out some challenging yet attainable goals to focus on. Focus on just a few at a time and remind yourself at the beginning of each day what you'll be working on. Then check back with this quiz in a few weeks. I'll bet you'll progress even more!

MOSTLY C'S

Master of good intentions.

Your goals are in sight! You fight off emotional and mindless eating most of the time, but you're human as well. Continue to be purposeful in your food selections, continue to pause before digging into your meal, and continue to review the pro tips throughout this book to help you tweak those few habits that need tweaking. Give yourself a pat on the back; your hard work is paying off, and you're doing a great job combating the call of cravings and coping with calories.

MOSTLY D'S

Willpower warrior.

Look at you, having a handle on how emotions can influence your health and wellness! You've cracked the code on how to eat with nutrition goals and good fueling in mind rather than use food to cope after a stressful day or as a tool to numb the pain of X, Y, or Z. You're mentally strong, mindful, and a stress-less eater. Now, if you're still not where you want to be nutritionally or physically, it may be time to take a look at total calorie intake (see the calculations in Determine Your Daily Energy Needs on pp. 66–71 and then take a deep dive into finding a macronutrient distribution (see Finding Your Macro Mix on pp. 72–75) that moves you in the right direction.

Your 90-Day Challenge

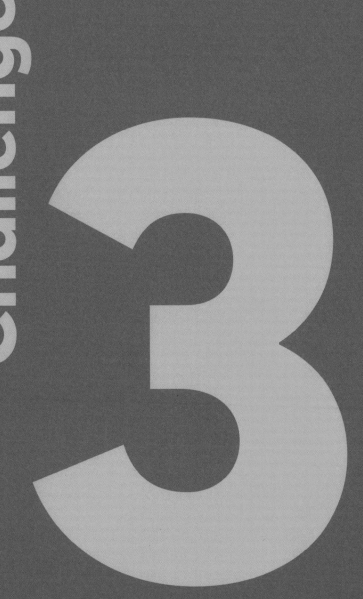

90 Days Starts Now

Problem-solving your daily diet requires you to detect fact from fiction. And oh! the opinions on how you should and shouldn't fuel and nourish your body. But what works for one person does not necessarily work for another. And a tactic or approach that doesn't work for the majority just might be what works for you. Nutrition needs to be unique because you are unique. I'm here to help you set a nutritional course specific to your goals. I will guide you as you grow in nutritional knowledge and confidence and make your way to a stronger, healthier you. In this section, you'll get the facts on nourishing nutrition, hear more advice from vetted experts, track what you eat each day, and ultimately figure out for yourself what belongs on your plate.

Are you feeling like you're in a good place with food? Making good decisions that nourish you and give you energy? Or are you feeling like you have some work to do? Maybe you're making what you believe to be the right choices most of the time but perhaps indulging more often than you think you should. Or maybe you know what the right choices are, but you simply need a reset to make those choices happen. Whatever your relationship with food, chances are you'd like to improve it. You've come to the right place. All of us have work to do. Me, you, even our Insta personalities who post amazing meals, but whose grocery carts in real life look a lot like ours. All of us can benefit from a better plate, a better connection with what fuels and nourishes us.

There might be people out there who have an amazing relationship with food, know the ins and outs of nutrition, and make the right food choice every damn time. This book is not for them . . . if they in fact exist. This journal is a 90-day playbook to change how you think and feel about food. **If you are ready to dig deep and make some lasting lifestyle changes and you are willing to track your stats along the way, then get ready to love the journey.**

Over the course of 90 days, as you use this guidebook and food journal, remember attitude is everything. Stay positive and believe in yourself. A better relationship with nutrition happens when you are confidently armed with nutrition knowledge and you have a plan to overcome those defeating *It won't work* thoughts. Inevitably, there will be days when you falter or feel like you've failed. Simply take a deep breath, pause, and reset. Be kind to yourself, and—most important—don't quit! Making positive changes takes work . . . and time. Don't stop journaling halfway through the 90 days. You need the whole 90 days to create a new habit and to build a new you, cell by cell by cell.

Over many years of practice, I've worked with countless individuals seeking a better relationship with food and those seeking better health and improved performance as a result of better choices. I've learned that my younger clients tend to listen more intently to the deafening cry of the taste buds rather than entertain conversations about longevity and cholesterol levels. I've learned that I'm not the only one who struggles to avoid emotional eating or mindless snacking out of boredom or stress. I've learned how to tweak a weight-loss warrior's macronutrient intake to keep energy levels high and hunger at bay so they can pursue their happy weight. And I've learned how to help elite athletes fuel their quest for the podium—in large part through my own experiences of how *not to fuel for a race*.

As a nutrition expert, I've gathered all of these experiences and placed them within the pages of this book. But, the most important

You do you.
Map your own course forward.

Some people will say
your choices are wrong,
or your goals are too bold.

Focus. Commit.
And prove them wrong.

thing I've come to know is that there are certain times in our lives that we are primed and ready to make changes. We have a clear head, seemingly limitless motivation, and the support we need to succeed. And then there are times in our lives when we are so stressed and busy that we simply are not equipped to change or to take on the task of eating better. No one knows your heart and mind better than you, so before you dive in, make sure that you are ready for this challenge. If not, that's okay too. When things calm down in your life and you have more time to focus on yourself and what's on your plate, this journal will be ready.

What you record in this journal is for you and you alone, so don't be embarrassed or ashamed about what you're eating. A day's intake is just a snapshot. It's not the be-all, end-all because better nutrition happens over time. Be gentle with yourself, and then *write it down!*

How to keep a food journal

1

Write down every single bite and sip that passes your lips. Capture the nutrient info by looking at a food's nutrition label, using the food tables on pp. 42–52 or by using online sources, like USDA's FoodData Central. After you do the work you can refer to earlier entries for the nutrition data of your favorite foods.

2

Write down your emotions, triggers, or any other aha moments that impact what you choose to eat and how you feel.

3

If you're training for an event, track your fueling. Note what works to fuel your performance as well as what doesn't agree with you. Massage your intake until you have a plan to rock race day.

4

Set goals for your daily diet and write them down. Keep an eye on this prize by using the habit tracker grids. By tracking your progress toward a new habit or goal, you'll be more motivated to stay the course.

5

Finally, take the time to plan for a better tomorrow. Summarize your weekly intake. What went well? Write down your plan to make next week better so over time, you continuously improve. If this sounds daunting, remember that anything worth having demands something of you.

Sample Journal Page

FOOD	CAL	CARBS (G)	FIBER (G)	PROT (G)	FAT (G)	OTHER
CHOBANI® YOGURT (PEACH)	110	16	<1	11	0	CALCIUM
COFFEE	5	0	0	0.5	0.5	
WHOLE MILK	50	2.5	0	2.5	2	CALCIUM
APPLE	100	24	4	0.5	0.5	

Hunger ☒ ⊟ ☒   Mood ☒ ⊟ ☒

HARD-BOILED EGG	155	1	0	13	11	LUTEIN
MOZZARELLA CHEESE STICK	70	1	0	6	5	CALCIUM
CRUDITÉS	65	5	5	4	3	
HUMMUS	51	4	2	2	3	

Hunger ☒ ☒ √   Mood ☒ ☒ √

NATURE'S BAKERY® FIG BAR	100	19	2	2	2.5	
BABY CARROTS	35	8				

Hangry   **Little hungry**   **Just fine**

Track hunger and mood around meals and snacks

Hunger ☒ ☒ √   Mood ☒ ⊟ √

BURGER	350	0	0	20	30	
BUN (WHITE)	125	22	1	4	2	
POTATO SALAD	285	34	0	4		
COLESLAW	105	4	1	0.5		

Bad   **Neutral**   **Good**

Hunger ☒ ⊟ √   Mood ☒ ⊟ √

DAILY TOTALS (G)	1,606	140.5	15	69	85	
MACROS (%)		35		17	48	

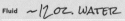

Fitness ELLIPTICAL + CORE STRENGTH

Duration 30 + 10 MIN.

Burn 200 + 50 CALORIES

Reflection RECOVERY DAY; WORKED ON LOWER ABS + BALANCE

Fuel FIG BARS, COFFEE, YOGURT

Pre-workout   Mid-workout   Post-workout

Fluid ~12 OZ. WATER   ← ☒ →

Fuel 30 G CARBS   ☒ ↔ ☒

Other 500 MG CALCIUM, OMEGA-3, MULTI   ☒ ↔ →

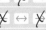

Pro tips on nailing your 90-day challenge

Journal as you go. It's difficult to recall what you ate at the end of the day. Write down *everything* you consume, as you eat it. And every bite counts.

Focus on portion size. Make good use of measuring cups, measuring spoons, food scales, and visual cues. It's common to underestimate how much food is actually consumed and portions tend to grow over time. So measure it out and note what the food looks like on your plate. Check back in periodically.

Cheat day? No problem. Write it down and give some extra thought to why you're choosing those foods. If it's because they are delicious, great. If you're eating them because you feel so freaking restricted during the week, it may be time to revisit your weekly meal plan.

Be consistent. Commit to tracking your diet and recording *every single bite*— whether it's a choice that makes you proud or a choice you're going to work on.

Details matter. Note the impact of seemingly inconsequential details. What time did you eat? . . . Did you go too long between meals and get hangry? Did you eat lunch simply because it was noon and not because you were actually hungry? Where did you eat? . . . Did the noise and excitement of happy hour drive you to choose unwisely? Did the calm and quiet of home lead you to choose better? What was your mood, your feelings before, during, and after? . . . Did your day-to-day dictate your intake, or did you consciously decide what's on your plate?

Plan ahead. And stick to the plan. You can even try writing out your meals and snacks *before you eat them* to see how each eating occasion will fit into your daily goals.

Metrics to Track Your Success

As humans, we live and die by certain metrics, and we give them the power to make or break our day. Nailed your goal weight? Best day ever! Failed to hit the gym? All feels lost. Depending on where we set the bar, all can feel lost more often than not.

Checking in on your progress and your pitfalls can be both helpful and cathartic. But don't rely on one number or one habit or one marker to tell you whether you're on the right track. And definitely resist the urge to track your metrics compulsively. Instead, thoughtfully consider the pieces of the puzzle that will help you to see the bigger picture. Focus on the metrics you need to improve in order to achieve better health, wellness, and comfort with what fuels you.

Every metric has its limitations, so I'll give you some advice on how to view them. Some metrics are tracked daily, others monthly or more infrequently, and together they show your progress, or evolution, to becoming the you that you are meant to be.

How you choose to define success is personal, but if you're not sure where to start, I'm happy to sound in: It involves more than the number on the scale. It's my hope that you will get to a place where you feel good about what's on your plate and how it nourishes you both physically and mentally. Here are some of the metrics you can use to measure your success.

Calorie Count

Why? Like it or not, your intake of calories drives the readout on many of these other metrics. Too many little bites of energy and you risk not meeting your body comp goals. Too few and you risk being injured or worn down and not meeting your fitness goals. You get the idea. Refer to Determine Your Daily Energy Needs, p. 66, to determine the calories you need to consume on a day-to-day basis. Commit to recording what you eat and be honest about calories consumed. Make the decision to improve from week to week. Look back over past weeks to see subtle changes that will get you closer to your goals. You've got this.

Check it: Daily. Every bite counts.

Macros Mix

Why? You need all three nutrients in the best ratios (see Finding Your Macro Mix on p. 72 for details) to optimally fuel your health and fitness goals. It's a balancing act. If you cut back too much on protein, you can end up feeling weak and broken down. Cut back on carbs and your body composition may improve, but your speed workouts feel like an uphill battle. The quality of the foods you choose makes a big difference in health and performance as well. If tracking the totals for each meal and tallying your ratio is more than you can commit to, track how many servings of each macronutrient you eat, at a bare minimum, to be sure you're getting the nutrition you need to fuel your day and your goals.

Check it: Daily. Every bite counts.

Weight

Why? Now that you know your goal weight or ideal weight (see p. 67 for the worksheet), it's time to move toward your goal. People who have lost weight and kept it off credit weight checks (at least once a week)

> **Keep moving toward a better tomorrow,**
>
> **and the metrics that matter will begin moving in the right direction.**

as a key metric of success. So get yourself a reliable, consistent scale. It needn't have fancy bells and whistles; it just needs to show you your progress over time and help keep you honest.

Check it: Once every one to two days, first thing in the morning after using the restroom. Don't waste your time stepping on the scale more often as weight can fluctuate due to food and fluid intake. And remember, this is just one piece of the puzzle. Don't give this number the power to make or break your day. You're worth more than the number on the scale.

Body Composition

Why? Your body composition goals (the percentage of fat mass and lean mass) need to take into account your performance and health goals. Extremes on either end of the spectrum can lead to poor health outcomes. In general, less fat and more muscle lead to better outcomes.

When the number on the scale seems stuck...

It's easy to get frustrated when you don't see the number on the scale change, but eating better and working out more consistently could actually be to blame. For example, eating more protein and adding in strength training can replace fat with lean muscle, so your body composition has changed even though your weight has not. You're still moving forward! Your pants will feel looser, and a reduction in abdominal fat can result in a reduction in chronic diseases. Weight is one simple metric and not the be-all, end-all, so if the number on the scale shows no love, look for other signs of good things.

Such as a faster 5K time, less stress on joints, higher metabolic burn, and even improved lab values. What's optimal for you depends on your physiology, your goals, and input from your health care provider.

Ideally, most men should aim to be within the range of 10 to 22 percent body fat; for women, the 20 to 32 percent range is considered satisfactory. Many athletes in heavy training or with a specific performance goal may want to aim lower. However, very low body fat percentages can have deleterious effects, so staying above 5 percent body fat for men and 12 percent for women is recommended. Depending upon the measurement method used, body fat percentages are not always spot on, so there will be a margin of error to consider.

How: Dual-energy X-ray absorptiometry (DEXA), underwater weighing, skinfold measurements, and bioelectrical impedance analysis (BIA) are all common tests that will give you your measurement. DEXA is the best but tends to be pricey. It's becoming more readily accessible, and most universities and hospitals have the ability to run this test. BIA is the test commonly used on home scales to supply a body fat percentage reading. It can be altered by hydration status, so just use it as a baseline and look for trends rather than put value on the actual number. As your training progresses and as you make improvements, checking in on your body comp can keep you motivated or steer you in a better direction.

Check it: On a home scale, check it weekly in the morning when you check your weight. Monitor the trend to see if you're making progress. If you have access to DEXA, the gold standard, aim to update your scans every three to six months.

Fitness Progress

Why? The nutrition changes you are making should positively impact your performance, so tracking the stats of your sweat session is key. Try monitoring the ease of identical workouts from week to week. Or use a 5K time trial to see if increasing protein for more muscle and better recovery is leading to aerobic improvement. Or maybe the pace you can sustain is faster thanks to better hydration, a more balanced intake of nutrients, or a different mix of calories.

Check it: Track workouts daily. Benchmark measurements—like the ones listed above—weekly or monthly.

Habits, Good or Bad

Why? Your habits not only drive you, they define you. Decide which habits matter and write them down, whether it's something along the lines of "eat five servings of veggies each day," or "drink 64 ounces of water," or "gain five pounds of muscle." On the other hand, you might have a bad habit you need to scrap altogether. Work on these habits daily, over the course of 30+ days. On average, most people agree that a habit followed over 60 days sticks. But the urge to give up on a habit often occurs after just a few weeks! Everyone is different—some people can make a habit stick in as little as three weeks, but others need months. As you select the habits to hone, do so with an honest understanding of your own nature. If you live for your morning coffee, going caffeine-free might do more harm than good. Exhausted by the time you get home from work? Then don't vow to work out every evening. Don't set yourself up for failure. Focus instead on personal growth and accept that what's perfect in one person's eyes may be flawed in your own and vice versa.

Check it: Daily. Stay consistent, but tweak your tracker goals from month to month, making small changes until you have reached a point where you shift from expending effort or restraint to simply acting without even thinking about it.

Map your way to a better tomorrow

Before you begin your 90-day challenge, take some time to reflect over recent weeks and months to better understand your current state of mind and the current state of your plate. Give some thought to the obstacles in your way. Think about the changes you want to make and the *why* driving those changes. Be honest. You know what success looks like for you.

Improving nutrition, health, and performance is all about balance. Here are some simple swaps I'm going to make in my daily diet.

Note: This could be a macronutrient such as carbs or fat or alcohol or a micronutrient such as sodium or iron.

Sometimes, less is more.
Going forward, I'll eat less:

My reasoning:

Sometimes, more is more.
Going forward, I'll eat more:

My reasoning:

If your plate is looking balanced, let's dig deeper: Is there anything you can do to further promote health and performance?

Looking back, my go-to pre-workout fuel has been:

Going forward, my go-to pre-workout fuel will become:

Looking back, I recover from a hard workout by:

Going forward, I'll recover by:

Map your way to a better tomorrow *(continued)*

I know when and why I make less-than-spectacular food choices.

Going forward, I'll make better choices by:

Looking back, I paid attention to the size of my portions:

☐ USUALLY/ALWAYS ☐ OFTEN ☐ SOMETIMES ☐ NEVER/RARELY

Going forward, I'll pay attention to portion sizes:

☐ USUALLY/ALWAYS ☐ OFTEN ☐ SOMETIMES ☐ NEVER/RARELY

Looking back, I've been tracking my calories and macros:

☐ USUALLY/ALWAYS ☐ OFTEN ☐ SOMETIMES ☐ NEVER/RARELY

Going forward, I'll track my calories and macros:

☐ USUALLY/ALWAYS ☐ OFTEN ☐ SOMETIMES ☐ NEVER/RARELY

Going forward, I'll become more consistent by:

My current macro mix:

% Carbs % Protein % Fat

My macro mix goal:

% Carbs % Protein % Fat

My reasoning:

My plan for consistency:

I know when and why I tend to make emotional eating choices.

Looking back, my emotions dictated my food intake:

☐ USUALLY/ALWAYS ☐ OFTEN ☐ SOMETIMES ☐ NEVER/RARELY

Going forward, my emotions will decide my food intake:

☐ USUALLY/ALWAYS ☐ OFTEN ☐ SOMETIMES ☐ NEVER/RARELY

Going forward, I'll prevent this by:

I'll work to limit my pattern of mindless eating:

☐ USUALLY/ALWAYS ☐ OFTEN ☐ SOMETIMES ☐ NEVER/RARELY

I know when I eat mindlessly and why:

Going forward, I'll prevent this by:

Now let's define what success looks like outside of the kitchen.

Looking back, I've exercised:

☐ MULTIPLE TIMES/DAY ☐ EVERY DAY ☐ A FEW TIMES/WEEK ☐ NEVER/RARELY

Going forward, I will exercise:

☐ MULTIPLE TIMES/DAY ☐ EVERY DAY ☐ A FEW TIMES/WEEK ☐ NEVER/RARELY

I know when and why I miss workouts:

Going forward, I'll prevent this by:

I am making these changes because:

SET YOUR INTENTION. Know where you hope to be in 90 days so you can confidently shout, *"I made it!"* upon arrival.

Monthly Habit Tracker

No doubt there are some habits you want to make and others you want to break.
Put them here and track your progress daily over the coming month.

		1	2	3	4	5	6	7	8	9	10	11	12	13	14	15	16
		17	18	19	20	21	22	23	24	25	26	27	28	29	30	31	

		1	2	3	4	5	6	7	8	9	10	11	12	13	14	15	16
		17	18	19	20	21	22	23	24	25	26	27	28	29	30	31	

		1	2	3	4	5	6	7	8	9	10	11	12	13	14	15	16
		17	18	19	20	21	22	23	24	25	26	27	28	29	30	31	

		1	2	3	4	5	6	7	8	9	10	11	12	13	14	15	16
		17	18	19	20	21	22	23	24	25	26	27	28	29	30	31	

		1	2	3	4	5	6	7	8	9	10	11	12	13	14	15	16
		17	18	19	20	21	22	23	24	25	26	27	28	29	30	31	

Week 1

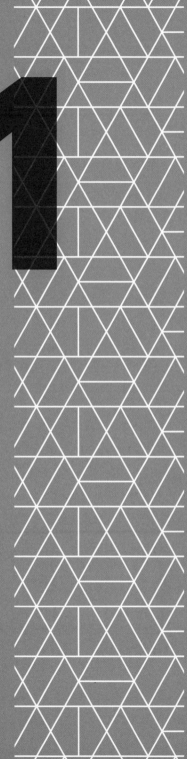

Believe in work

Think back to a time when you felt great and looked amazing. Chances are good that the last time you were glowing with self-confidence (and maybe your jeans fit perfectly too), you were putting in some sweat equity. Never forget that success like this takes work. Better health and performance call for some time at the gym, some extra effort and intention in the kitchen, and willpower at the dining table. It's not easy. Nothing worth having is. But when you work for something you want, your work becomes a habit. And eventually, it becomes less about doing the work and more about doing something you believe in—something you are passionate about. You grow accustomed to setting your alarm clock because you *want* to rise early and hustle right before work. You become the coworker who meal preps on the weekend and brings in balanced lunches instead of grabbing fast food. You become the person who politely declines a second helping most of the time! Reaching your goals mandates you put in the work.

FOOD	CAL	CARBS (G)	FIBER (G)	PROT (G)	FAT (G)	OTHER

Hunger ☒ ☐ ☑   Mood ☒ ☐ ☑

Hunger ☒ ☐ ☑   Mood ☒ ☐ ☑

Hunger ☒ ☐ ☑   Mood ☒ ☐ ☑

Hunger ☒ ☐ ☑   Mood ☒ ☐ ☑

DAILY TOTALS (G)

MACROS (%)

1

Fitness

Duration

Burn

Reflection

Fuel

Fluid ← ↔ →

Fuel ← ↔ →

Other ← ↔ →

FOOD		CAL	CARBS (G)	FIBER (G)	PROT (G)	FAT (G)	OTHER

Hunger ⊠ ⊟ ☑ Mood ⊠ ⊟ ☑

Hunger ⊠ ⊟ ☑ Mood ⊠ ⊟ ☑

Hunger ⊠ ⊟ ☑ Mood ⊠ ⊟ ☑

Hunger ⊠ ⊟ ☑ Mood ⊠ ⊟ ☑

DAILY TOTALS (G)

MACROS (%)

2

Fitness

Duration

Burn

Reflection

Fuel

Fluid ← ↔ →

Fuel ← ↔ →

Other ← ↔ →

DO THE WORK

FOOD	CAL	CARBS (G)	FIBER (G)	PROT (G)	FAT (G)	OTHER

Hunger ☒ ☐ ☑   Mood ☒ ☐ ☑

Hunger ☒ ☐ ☑   Mood ☒ ☐ ☑

Hunger ☒ ☐ ☑   Mood ☒ ☐ ☑

Hunger ☒ ☐ ☑   Mood ☒ ☐ ☑

DAILY TOTALS (G)

MACROS (%)

3

Fitness

Duration

Burn

Reflection

Fuel

Fluid ← ↔ →

Fuel ← ↔ →

Other ← ↔ →

FOOD	CAL	CARBS (G)	FIBER (G)	PROT (G)	FAT (G)	OTHER

Hunger ☒ ☐ ☑   Mood ☒ ☐ ☑

Hunger ☒ ☐ ☑   Mood ☒ ☐ ☑

Hunger ☒ ☐ ☑   Mood ☒ ☐ ☑

Hunger ☒ ☐ ☑   Mood ☒ ☐ ☑

DAILY TOTALS (G)

MACROS (%)

4

Fitness

Duration

Burn

Reflection

Fuel

Fluid   ← ↔ →

Fuel   ← ↔ →

Other   ← ↔ →

DO THE WORK

FOOD		CAL	CARBS (G)	FIBER (G)	PROT (G)	FAT (G)	OTHER

Hunger ☒ ☐ ☑   Mood ☒ ☐ ☑

Hunger ☒ ☐ ☑   Mood ☒ ☐ ☑

Hunger ☒ ☐ ☑   Mood ☒ ☐ ☑

Hunger ☒ ☐ ☑   Mood ☒ ☐ ☑

DAILY TOTALS (G)

MACROS (%)

5

Fitness

Duration

Burn

Reflection

Fuel

Fluid   ← ↔ →

Fuel   ← ↔ →

Other   ← ↔ →

FOOD		CAL	CARBS (G)	FIBER (G)	PROT (G)	FAT (G)	OTHER

Hunger ⊠ ⊟ ☑ Mood ⊠ ⊟ ☑

Hunger ⊠ ⊟ ☑ Mood ⊠ ⊟ ☑

Hunger ⊠ ⊟ ☑ Mood ⊠ ⊟ ☑

Hunger ⊠ ⊟ ☑ Mood ⊠ ⊟ ☑

DAILY TOTALS (G)

MACROS (%)

6

Fitness

Duration

Burn

Reflection

Fuel

Fluid ← ↔ →

Fuel ← ↔ →

Other ← ↔ →

DO THE WORK

FOOD				CAL	CARBS (G)	FIBER (G)	PROT (G)	FAT (G)	OTHER

Hunger ☒ ☐— ☐√   Mood ☒ ☐— ☐√

Hunger ☒ ☐— ☐√   Mood ☒ ☐— ☐√

Hunger ☒ ☐— ☐√   Mood ☒ ☐— ☐√

Hunger ☒ ☐— ☐√   Mood ☒ ☐— ☐√

DAILY TOTALS (G)

MACROS (%)

7

Fitness

Duration

Burn

Reflection

Fuel

Fluid ← ↔ →

Fuel ← ↔ →

Other ← ↔ →

Week 1 Review

Average weekly blend

macros

% Carbs   % Protein   % Fat

Wins & losses

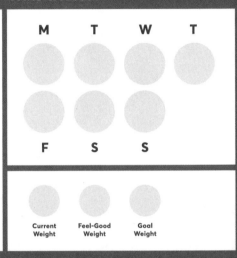

| M | T | W | T |

| F | S | S |

Current Weight   Feel-Good Weight   Goal Weight

For a better tomorrow

Fitness   ☒ ☐ ☑

Next week I will . . .

⬆

➡

Fuel   ☒ ☐ ☑

Next week I will . . .

⬆

➡

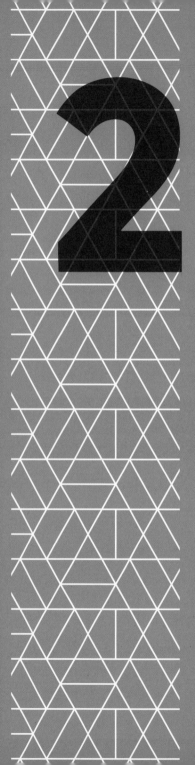

Week 2

Find balance

Mild and occasional hunger is okay in the fight for weight loss. I know, mind blown, right?! The hormonal signals that prompt you to eat are triggered when there's a calorie deficit, which is a good thing when it comes to weight loss, and these signals are necessary to get the metabolism fired up. But regardless of your health and performance goals, you don't need to impose a weeklong fast where you don't eat between the hours of 8:00 a.m. and 8:00 p.m. (Or was it 7:00 a.m. to 3:00 p.m.? Or 2:00 a.m. to 9:00 p.m.?), or never enjoy dessert, ever. Certainly, some food choices are better choices than others, and you don't need to eat every two hours in order to survive, but you don't need an expert to tell you that! To be successful long-term, constant deprivation or promotion of painful practices to induce unsustainable weight loss won't work. Instead, try eating purposeful portions of mindful meals and snacks throughout the day and make every single bite do something for your health in addition to doing something for your taste buds.

FOOD		CAL	CARBS (G)	FIBER (G)	PROT (G)	FAT (G)	OTHER

Hunger ☒ ☐ ☑   Mood ☒ ☐ ☑

Hunger ☒ ☐ ☑   Mood ☒ ☐ ☑

Hunger ☒ ☐ ☑   Mood ☒ ☐ ☑

Hunger ☒ ☐ ☑   Mood ☒ ☐ ☑

DAILY TOTALS (G)

MACROS (%)

8

Fitness

Duration

Burn

Reflection

Fuel

Fluid   ← ↔ →

Fuel   ← ↔ →

Other   ← ↔ →

PROGRESS, NOT PERFECTION

FOOD		CAL	CARBS (G)	FIBER (G)	PROT (G)	FAT (G)	OTHER
		Hunger ☒ — ☑			Mood ☒ — ☑		
		Hunger ☒ — ☑			Mood ☒ — ☑		
		Hunger ☒ — ☑			Mood ☒ — ☑		
		Hunger ☒ — ☑			Mood ☒ — ☑		
DAILY TOTALS (G)							
MACROS (%)							

9

Fitness

Duration

Burn

Reflection

Fuel

Fluid ← ↔ →

Fuel ← ↔ →

Other ← ↔ →

FOOD	CAL	CARBS (G)	FIBER (G)	PROT (G)

Hunger ☒ ☐ ☑

FOOD	CAL	CARBS (G)	FIBER (G)	PROT (G)

Hunger ☒ ☐ ☑

Hunger ☒ ☐ ☑

Hunger ☒ ☐ ☑

DAILY TOTALS (G)

MACROS (%)

10

Fitness

Duration

Burn

Reflection

Fuel

Fluid ←

Fuel ←

Other ←

PROGRESS, NOT PERFEC

	CAL	CARBS (G)	FIBER (G)	PROT (G)	FAT (G)	OTHER
						Hunger ☒ ☐ ☑ Mood ☒ ☐ ☑
						Hunger ☒ ☐ ☑ Mood ☒ ☐ ☑
						Hunger ☒ ☐ ☑ Mood ☒ ☐ ☑
						Hunger ☒ ☐ ☑ Mood ☒ ☐ ☑
DAILY TOTALS (G)						
MACROS (%)						

11

Fitness

Duration

Burn

Reflection

Fuel

Fluid   ← ↔ →

Fuel   ← ↔ →

Other   ← ↔ →

FOOD	CAL	CARBS (G)	FIBER (G)	PROT (G)	FAT (G)	OTHER

Hunger × — √   Mood × — √

Hunger × — √   Mood × — √

Hunger × — √   Mood × — √

Hunger × — √   Mood × — √

DAILY TOTALS (G)

MACROS (%)

12

Fitness

Duration

Burn

Reflection

Fuel

Fluid ← ↔ →

Fuel ← ↔ →

Other ← ↔ →

PROGRESS, NOT PERFECTION

FOOD	CAL	CARBS (G)	FIBER (G)	PROT (G)	FAT (G)	OTHER

Hunger ☒ — ✓   Mood ☒ — ✓

Hunger ☒ — ✓   Mood ☒ — ✓

Hunger ☒ — ✓   Mood ☒ — ✓

Hunger ☒ — ✓   Mood ☒ — ✓

DAILY TOTALS (G)

MACROS (%)

13

Fitness

Duration

Burn

Reflection

Fuel

Fluid ← ↔ →

Fuel ← ↔ →

Other ← ↔ →

FOOD		CAL	CARBS (G)	FIBER (G)	PROT (G)	FAT (G)	OTHER
				Hunger ☒ ☐ ☑		Mood ☒ ☐ ☑	
				Hunger ☒ ☐ ☑		Mood ☒ ☐ ☑	
				Hunger ☒ ☐ ☑		Mood ☒ ☐ ☑	
				Hunger ☒ ☐ ☑		Mood ☒ ☐ ☑	
DAILY TOTALS (G)							
MACROS (%)							

14

Fitness

Duration

Burn

Reflection

Fuel

Fluid ← ↔ →

Fuel ← ↔ →

Other ← ↔ →

PROGRESS, NOT PERFECTION

Week 2 Review

Average weekly blend

macros

% Carbs   % Protein   % Fat

Wins & losses

M	T	W	T

F	S	S

Current Weight   Feel-Good Weight   Goal Weight

For a better tomorrow

Fitness   ☒ ☐ ☑

⇧

Next week I will . . .

⇨

Fuel   ☒ ☐ ☑

⇧

Next week I will . . .

⇨

Week 3

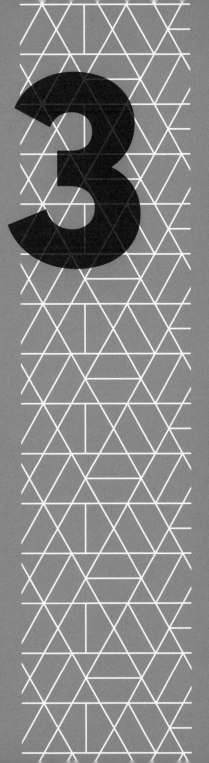

Math matters

Finding your feel-good weight doesn't happen as a result of some hyped ingredient in a pricey pill or any other form of snake oil that you might find in the dark corners of a weight-loss site. Millions of dollars are made on seems-too-good-to-be-true weight-loss fixes, but the real solution is simple, sustainable, and affordable. Truly effective solutions work because they remove empty calories, inspire metabolic changes, and create a calorie deficit. Whether that calorie deficit comes from a removal of carbs, or fat, or protein . . . or donuts or beer, it stems from removing whatever culprit might be holding you back. Sure, there are nuances to every diet and every macro, but if you focus first on calories in being less than calories out, you'll be on the path toward your health and performance goals.

FOOD	CAL	CARBS (G)	FIBER (G)	PROT (G)	FAT (G)	OTHER
	Hunger ☒ ☐ ☑			Mood ☒ ☐ ☑		
	Hunger ☒ ☐ ☑			Mood ☒ ☐ ☑		
	Hunger ☒ ☐ ☑			Mood ☒ ☐ ☑		
	Hunger ☒ ☐ ☑			Mood ☒ ☐ ☑		
DAILY TOTALS (G)						
MACROS (%)						

15

Fitness

Duration

Burn

Reflection

Fuel

Fluid ← ↔ →

Fuel ← ↔ →

Other ← ↔ →

FOOD	CAL	CARBS (G)	FIBER (G)	PROT (G)	FAT (G)	OTHER

Hunger ☒ ☐ ☑   Mood ☒ ☐ ☑

Hunger ☒ ☐ ☑   Mood ☒ ☐ ☑

Hunger ☒ ☐ ☑   Mood ☒ ☐ ☑

Hunger ☒ ☐ ☑   Mood ☒ ☐ ☑

DAILY TOTALS (G)

MACROS (%)

16

Fitness

Duration

Burn

Reflection

Fuel

Fluid ← ↔ →

Fuel ← ↔ →

Other ← ↔ →

DO THE MATH

FOOD	CAL	CARBS (G)	FIBER (G)	PROT (G)	FAT (G)	OTHER

Hunger ☒ ☐ ☑   Mood ☒ ☐ ☑

Hunger ☒ ☐ ☑   Mood ☒ ☐ ☑

Hunger ☒ ☐ ☑   Mood ☒ ☐ ☑

Hunger ☒ ☐ ☑   Mood ☒ ☐ ☑

DAILY TOTALS (G)

MACROS (%)

17

Fitness

Duration

Burn

Reflection

Fuel

Fluid ← ↔ →

Fuel ← ↔ →

Other ← ↔ →

FOOD		CAL	CARBS (G)	FIBER (G)	PROT (G)	FAT (G)	OTHER

Hunger ☒ ☐ ☑ Mood ☒ ☐ ☑

Hunger ☒ ☐ ☑ Mood ☒ ☐ ☑

Hunger ☒ ☐ ☑ Mood ☒ ☐ ☑

Hunger ☒ ☐ ☑ Mood ☒ ☐ ☑

DAILY TOTALS (G)

MACROS (%)

18

Fitness

Duration

Burn

Reflection

Fuel

Fluid ← ↔ →

Fuel ← ↔ →

Other ← ↔ →

DO THE MATH

FOOD	CAL	CARBS (G)	FIBER (G)	PROT (G)	FAT (G)	OTHER

Hunger ☒ ☐ ☑   Mood ☒ ☐ ☑

Hunger ☒ ☐ ☑   Mood ☒ ☐ ☑

Hunger ☒ ☐ ☑   Mood ☒ ☐ ☑

Hunger ☒ ☐ ☑   Mood ☒ ☐ ☑

DAILY TOTALS (G)

MACROS (%)

19

Fitness

Duration

Burn

Reflection

Fuel

Fluid   ← ↔ →

Fuel   ← ↔ →

Other   ← ↔ →

FOOD	CAL	CARBS (G)	FIBER (G)	PROT (G)	FAT (G)	OTHER

Hunger × − √   Mood × − √

Hunger × − √   Mood × − √

Hunger × − √   Mood × − √

Hunger × − √   Mood × − √

DAILY TOTALS (G)

MACROS (%)

20

Fitness

Duration

Burn

Reflection

Fuel

Fluid   ← ↔ →

Fuel   ← ↔ →

Other   ← ↔ →

DO THE MATH

FOOD	CAL	CARBS (G)	FIBER (G)	PROT (G)	FAT (G)	OTHER

Hunger ☒ ⊟ ☑   Mood ☒ ⊟ ☑

Hunger ☒ ⊟ ☑   Mood ☒ ⊟ ☑

Hunger ☒ ⊟ ☑   Mood ☒ ⊟ ☑

Hunger ☒ ⊟ ☑   Mood ☒ ⊟ ☑

DAILY TOTALS (G)

MACROS (%)

21

Fitness

Duration

Burn

Reflection

Fuel

Fluid   ← ↔ →

Fuel   ← ↔ →

Other   ← ↔ →

Average weekly blend

macros

% Carbs   % Protein   % Fat

Wins & losses

M	T	W	T

F	S	S

Current
Weight

Feel-Good
Weight

Goal
Weight

For a better tomorrow

Fitness   ☒ ⊟ ☑

⇧

Next week I will . . .

⇨

Fuel   ☒ ⊟ ☑

⇧

Next week I will . . .

⇨

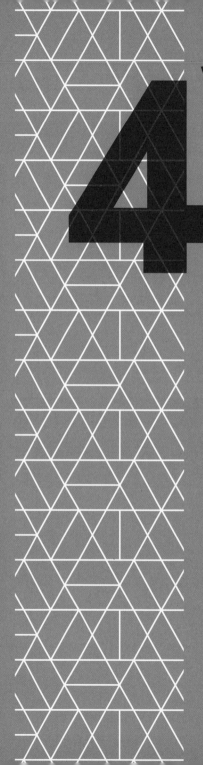

Week 4

Build a better plate

Countless diets have been derailed by empty calories from refined grains, sugar fixes, and carb-rich foods devoid of the staying power that comes with satiating protein-rich foods and satisfying high-fat foods. Which is why your goal this week is to think twice before you dine à la carb and miss out on protein and fat! If you're looking to get lean and mean, you need to opt for a diet that is calorie controlled yet balanced; crap carbs can be eliminated without worrying about lost nutrients. Better choices come from whole foods that do more than just provide quick energy—grab nutrient-dense whole-grain, fruit, and vegetable sources and low-fat dairy as these contain vitamins, minerals, fiber, phytonutrients, and other health benefits.

FOOD	CAL	CARBS (G)	FIBER (G)	PROT (G)	FAT (G)	OTHER

Hunger ☒ ☐ ☑ Mood ☒ ☐ ☑

Hunger ☒ ☐ ☑ Mood ☒ ☐ ☑

Hunger ☒ ☐ ☑ Mood ☒ ☐ ☑

Hunger ☒ ☐ ☑ Mood ☒ ☐ ☑

DAILY TOTALS (G)

MACROS (%)

22

Fitness

Duration

Burn

Reflection

Fuel

Fluid ← ↔ →

Fuel ← ↔ →

Other ← ↔ →

BUILD A BETTER YOU

FOOD	CAL	CARBS (G)	FIBER (G)	PROT (G)	FAT (G)	OTHER

Hunger ☒ ☐ ☑ Mood ☒ ☐ ☑

Hunger ☒ ☐ ☑ Mood ☒ ☐ ☑

Hunger ☒ ☐ ☑ Mood ☒ ☐ ☑

Hunger ☒ ☐ ☑ Mood ☒ ☐ ☑

DAILY TOTALS (G)

MACROS (%)

23

Fitness

Duration

Burn

Reflection

Fuel

Fluid ← ↔ →

Fuel ← ↔ →

Other ← ↔ →

FOOD	CAL	CARBS (G)	FIBER (G)	PROT (G)	FAT (G)	OTHER

Hunger ☒ ☐ ☑ Mood ☒ ☐ ☑

Hunger ☒ ☐ ☑ Mood ☒ ☐ ☑

Hunger ☒ ☐ ☑ Mood ☒ ☐ ☑

Hunger ☒ ☐ ☑ Mood ☒ ☐ ☑

DAILY TOTALS (G)

MACROS (%)

24

Fitness

Duration

Burn

Reflection

Fuel

Fluid ← ↔ →

Fuel ← ↔ →

Other ← ↔ →

BUILD A BETTER YOU

FOOD	CAL	CARBS (G)	FIBER (G)	PROT (G)	FAT (G)	OTHER

Hunger ☒ ☐ ☑   Mood ☒ ☐ ☑

Hunger ☒ ☐ ☑   Mood ☒ ☐ ☑

Hunger ☒ ☐ ☑   Mood ☒ ☐ ☑

Hunger ☒ ☐ ☑   Mood ☒ ☐ ☑

DAILY TOTALS (G)

MACROS (%)

25

Fitness

Duration

Burn

Reflection

Fuel

Fluid

Fuel

Other

FOOD	CAL	CARBS (G)	FIBER (G)	PROT (G)	FAT (G)	OTHER

Hunger ☒ ☐ ☑ Mood ☒ ☐ ☑

Hunger ☒ ☐ ☑ Mood ☒ ☐ ☑

Hunger ☒ ☐ ☑ Mood ☒ ☐ ☑

Hunger ☒ ☐ ☑ Mood ☒ ☐ ☑

DAILY TOTALS (G)

MACROS (%)

26

Fitness

Duration

Burn

Reflection

Fuel

Fluid ← ↔ →

Fuel ← ↔ →

Other ← ↔ →

BUILD A BETTER YOU

FOOD	CAL	CARBS (G)	FIBER (G)	PROT (G)	FAT (G)	OTHER

Hunger ☒ ☐ ☑   Mood ☒ ☐ ☑

Hunger ☒ ☐ ☑   Mood ☒ ☐ ☑

Hunger ☒ ☐ ☑   Mood ☒ ☐ ☑

Hunger ☒ ☐ ☑   Mood ☒ ☐ ☑

DAILY TOTALS (G)

MACROS (%)

27

Fitness

Duration

Burn

Reflection

Fuel

Fluid ← ↔ →

Fuel ← ↔ →

Other ← ↔ →

FOOD		CAL	CARBS (G)	FIBER (G)	PROT (G)	FAT (G)	OTHER

Hunger ☒ ☐ ☑ Mood ☒ ☐ ☑

Hunger ☒ ☐ ☑ Mood ☒ ☐ ☑

Hunger ☒ ☐ ☑ Mood ☒ ☐ ☑

Hunger ☒ ☐ ☑ Mood ☒ ☐ ☑

DAILY TOTALS (G)

MACROS (%)

28

Fitness

Duration

Burn

Reflection

Fuel

Fluid ← ↔ →

Fuel ← ↔ →

Other ← ↔ →

BUILD A BETTER YOU

Week 4 Review

Average weekly blend

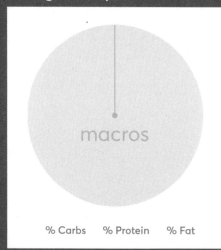

macros

% Carbs   % Protein   % Fat

Wins & losses

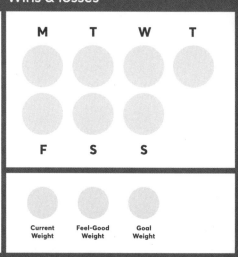

M   T   W   T

F   S   S

Current   Feel-Good   Goal
Weight   Weight   Weight

For a better tomorrow

Fitness   ☒ ⊟ ☑

⇧

Next week I will . . .

⇨

Fuel   ☒ ⊟ ☑

⇧

Next week I will . . .

⇨

Monthly Habit Tracker

No doubt there are some habits you want to make and others you want to break.
Put them here and track your progress daily over the coming month.

	1	2	3	4	5	6	7	8	9	10	11	12	13	14	15	16
	17	18	19	20	21	22	23	24	25	26	27	28	29	30	31	

	1	2	3	4	5	6	7	8	9	10	11	12	13	14	15	16
	17	18	19	20	21	22	23	24	25	26	27	28	29	30	31	

	1	2	3	4	5	6	7	8	9	10	11	12	13	14	15	16
	17	18	19	20	21	22	23	24	25	26	27	28	29	30	31	

	1	2	3	4	5	6	7	8	9	10	11	12	13	14	15	16
	17	18	19	20	21	22	23	24	25	26	27	28	29	30	31	

	1	2	3	4	5	6	7	8	9	10	11	12	13	14	15	16
	17	18	19	20	21	22	23	24	25	26	27	28	29	30	31	

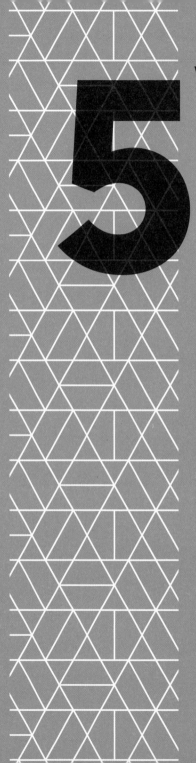

Week

5

Don't reinvent the wheel

Years of research prove that there are clear practices needed to shed weight and keep it off. Consider the National Weight Control Registry (NWCR), the largest prospective investigation of long-term successful weight loss. The NWCR tracks more than 10,000 individuals who have shed weight (an average of 66 pounds) and kept it off for more than 5.5 years, debunking the myth that long-term weight loss is impossible. Here's what these success stories share in common: a reduced-calorie diet that starts with breakfast, a weekly weigh-in, fewer hours sitting (and staring at media!), and one hour of exercise a day. There's no magic potion, no secret sauce, no supplements that will get you to a place of sustainable, happy eating and happy weight. Overnight weight loss is a short-term fix, and when you run out of the strength to stay on a detox or you simply can't stomach another meal of all-meat-all-the-time, you'll be right back where you started. So focus instead on purposeful choices and habits that lead to calories in being less than calories out and finding opportunities for plenty of movement throughout the day. No snake oil needed.

FOOD						CAL	CARBS (G)	FIBER (G)	PROT (G)	FAT (G)	OTHER

Hunger ☒ ☐ ☑   Mood ☒ ☐ ☑

Hunger ☒ ☐ ☑   Mood ☒ ☐ ☑

Hunger ☒ ☐ ☑   Mood ☒ ☐ ☑

Hunger ☒ ☐ ☑   Mood ☒ ☐ ☑

DAILY TOTALS (G)

MACROS (%)

29

Fitness

Duration

Burn

Reflection

Fuel

Fluid ← ↔ →

Fuel ← ↔ →

Other ← ↔ →

REINVENT YOURSELF

FOOD	CAL	CARBS (G)	FIBER (G)	PROT (G)	FAT (G)	OTHER

Hunger ☒ ☐− ☐✓   Mood ☒ ☐− ☐✓

Hunger ☒ ☐− ☐✓   Mood ☒ ☐− ☐✓

Hunger ☒ ☐− ☐✓   Mood ☒ ☐− ☐✓

Hunger ☒ ☐− ☐✓   Mood ☒ ☐− ☐✓

DAILY TOTALS (G)

MACROS (%)

30

Fitness

Duration

Burn

Reflection

Fuel

Fluid ← ↔ →

Fuel ← ↔ →

Other ← ↔ →

FOOD		CAL	CARBS (G)	FIBER (G)	PROT (G)	FAT (G)	OTHER

Hunger ☒ ☐ ☑   Mood ☒ ☐ ☑

Hunger ☒ ☐ ☑   Mood ☒ ☐ ☑

Hunger ☒ ☐ ☑   Mood ☒ ☐ ☑

Hunger ☒ ☐ ☑   Mood ☒ ☐ ☑

DAILY TOTALS (G)

MACROS (%)

31

Fitness

Duration

Burn

Reflection

Fuel

Fluid   ← ↔ →

Fuel   ← ↔ →

Other   ← ↔ →

REINVENT YOURSELF

FOOD	CAL	CARBS (G)	FIBER (G)	PROT (G)	FAT (G)	OTHER

Hunger ☒ ☐ ☑   Mood ☒ ☐ ☑

Hunger ☒ ☐ ☑   Mood ☒ ☐ ☑

Hunger ☒ ☐ ☑   Mood ☒ ☐ ☑

Hunger ☒ ☐ ☑   Mood ☒ ☐ ☑

DAILY TOTALS (G)

MACROS (%)

32

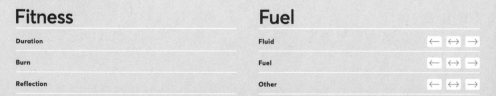

Fitness

Duration

Burn

Reflection

Fuel

Fluid   ← ↔ →

Fuel   ← ↔ →

Other   ← ↔ →

FOOD	CAL	CARBS (G)	FIBER (G)	PROT (G)	FAT (G)	OTHER

Hunger ☒ ☐ ☑   Mood ☒ ☐ ☑

Hunger ☒ ☐ ☑   Mood ☒ ☐ ☑

Hunger ☒ ☐ ☑   Mood ☒ ☐ ☑

Hunger ☒ ☐ ☑   Mood ☒ ☐ ☑

DAILY TOTALS (G)

MACROS (%)

33

Fitness

Duration

Burn

Reflection

Fuel

Fluid ← ↔ →

Fuel ← ↔ →

Other ← ↔ →

REINVENT YOURSELF

FOOD	CAL	CARBS (G)	FIBER (G)	PROT (G)	FAT (G)	OTHER

Hunger ☒ ☐ ☑   Mood ☒ ☐ ☑

Hunger ☒ ☐ ☑   Mood ☒ ☐ ☑

Hunger ☒ ☐ ☑   Mood ☒ ☐ ☑

Hunger ☒ ☐ ☑   Mood ☒ ☐ ☑

DAILY TOTALS (G)

MACROS (%)

34

Fitness

Duration

Burn

Reflection

Fuel

Fluid   ← ↔ →

Fuel   ← ↔ →

Other   ← ↔ →

FOOD				CAL	CARBS (G)	FIBER (G)	PROT (G)	FAT (G)	OTHER

Hunger ☒ ☐ ☑   Mood ☒ ☐ ☑

Hunger ☒ ☐ ☑   Mood ☒ ☐ ☑

Hunger ☒ ☐ ☑   Mood ☒ ☐ ☑

Hunger ☒ ☐ ☑   Mood ☒ ☐ ☑

DAILY TOTALS (G)

MACROS (%)

35

Fitness

Duration

Burn

Reflection

Fuel

Fluid ← ↔ →

Fuel ← ↔ →

Other ← ↔ →

REINVENT YOURSELF

Week 5 Review

Average weekly blend

macros

% Carbs   % Protein   % Fat

Wins & losses

M	T	W	T

F   **S**   **S**

Current
Weight

Feel-Good
Weight

Goal
Weight

For a better tomorrow

Fitness

☒ ▢ ☑

Next week I will . . .

Fuel

☒ ▢ ☑

Next week I will . . .

Week 6

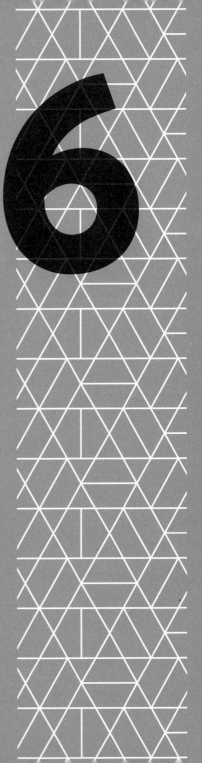

Cut out the crap

Did you know that a high intake of added sugar can be linked to a host of chronic diseases? Inflammation. Tooth decay. Obesity. Cravings. Foods that are high in sugar can create a drive to consume *more* foods that are high in sugar. Which doesn't help when you're trying to cut calories and build willpower. The World Health Organization recommends we cut back to no more than 5 percent of our calories from added sugar. For most of us, this is less than 25 grams a day. But foods that are high in sugar often taste delicious, probably because humans are hardwired to seek rapid energy and thus survive. This week, flex your willpower and walk away from foods that are high in added sugar. It will take some resolve, but over time, your self-discipline muscles will grow strong enough to stare down the call of your sweet tooth. I promise.

FOOD	CAL	CARBS (G)	FIBER (G)	PROT (G)	FAT (G)	OTHER

Hunger ☒ ☐ ☑   Mood ☒ ☐ ☑

Hunger ☒ ☐ ☑   Mood ☒ ☐ ☑

Hunger ☒ ☐ ☑   Mood ☒ ☐ ☑

Hunger ☒ ☐ ☑   Mood ☒ ☐ ☑

DAILY TOTALS (G)

MACROS (%)

36

Fitness

Duration

Burn

Reflection

Fuel

Fluid   ← ↔ →

Fuel   ← ↔ →

Other   ← ↔ →

FOOD		CAL	CARBS (G)	FIBER (G)	PROT (G)	FAT (G)	OTHER

Hunger ☒ ▭ ☑ Mood ☒ ▭ ☑

Hunger ☒ ▭ ☑ Mood ☒ ▭ ☑

Hunger ☒ ▭ ☑ Mood ☒ ▭ ☑

Hunger ☒ ▭ ☑ Mood ☒ ▭ ☑

DAILY TOTALS (G)

MACROS (%)

37

Fitness

Duration

Burn

Reflection

Fuel

Fluid ← ↔ →

Fuel ← ↔ →

Other ← ↔ →

FOOD	CAL	CARBS (G)	FIBER (G)	PROT (G)	FAT (G)	OTHER

Hunger ☒ ☐ ☑   Mood ☒ ☐ ☑

Hunger ☒ ☐ ☑   Mood ☒ ☐ ☑

Hunger ☒ ☐ ☑   Mood ☒ ☐ ☑

Hunger ☒ ☐ ☑   Mood ☒ ☐ ☑

DAILY TOTALS (G)

MACROS (%)

38

Fitness

Duration

Burn

Reflection

Fuel

Fluid ← ↔ →

Fuel ← ↔ →

Other ← ↔ →

FOOD		CAL	CARBS (G)	FIBER (G)	PROT (G)	FAT (G)	OTHER
				Hunger ☒ ☐ ☑	Mood ☒ ☐ ☑		
				Hunger ☒ ☐ ☑	Mood ☒ ☐ ☑		
				Hunger ☒ ☐ ☑	Mood ☒ ☐ ☑		
				Hunger ☒ ☐ ☑	Mood ☒ ☐ ☑		
DAILY TOTALS (G)							
MACROS (%)							

39

Fitness

Duration

Burn

Reflection

Fuel

Fluid ← ↔ →

Fuel ← ↔ →

Other ← ↔ →

FLEX YOUR WILLPOWER

FOOD		CAL	CARBS (G)	FIBER (G)	PROT (G)	FAT (G)	OTHER

Hunger ☒ ☐ ☑ Mood ☒ ☐ ☑

Hunger ☒ ☐ ☑ Mood ☒ ☐ ☑

Hunger ☒ ☐ ☑ Mood ☒ ☐ ☑

Hunger ☒ ☐ ☑ Mood ☒ ☐ ☑

DAILY TOTALS (G)

MACROS (%)

40

Fitness

Duration

Burn

Reflection

Fuel

Fluid ← ↔ →

Fuel ← ↔ →

Other ← ↔ →

FOOD	CAL	CARBS (G)	FIBER (G)	PROT (G)	FAT (G)	OTHER

Hunger ☒ ☐ ☑ Mood ☒ ☐ ☑

Hunger ☒ ☐ ☑ Mood ☒ ☐ ☑

Hunger ☒ ☐ ☑ Mood ☒ ☐ ☑

Hunger ☒ ☐ ☑ Mood ☒ ☐ ☑

DAILY TOTALS (G)

MACROS (%)

41

Fitness

Duration

Burn

Reflection

Fuel

Fluid ← ↔ →

Fuel ← ↔ →

Other ← ↔ →

FLEX YOUR WILLPOWER

FOOD	CAL	CARBS (G)	FIBER (G)	PROT (G)	FAT (G)	OTHER

Hunger ⊠ — ✓   Mood ⊠ — ✓

Hunger ⊠ — ✓   Mood ⊠ — ✓

Hunger ⊠ — ✓   Mood ⊠ — ✓

Hunger ⊠ — ✓   Mood ⊠ — ✓

DAILY TOTALS (G)

MACROS (%)

42

Fitness

Duration

Burn

Reflection

Fuel

Fluid ← ↔ →

Fuel ← ↔ →

Other ← ↔ →

Week 6 Review

Average weekly blend

macros

% Carbs   % Protein   % Fat

Wins & losses

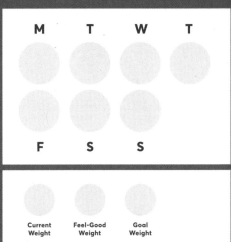

M	T	W	T

F   S   S

Current Weight   Feel-Good Weight   Goal Weight

For a better tomorrow

Fitness   ☒ ☐ ☑

⇧

Next week I will . . .

⇨

Fuel   ☒ ☐ ☑

⇧

Next week I will . . .

⇨

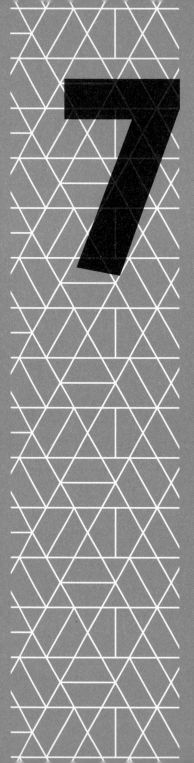

Week 7

Believe in filling fiber

When you consider the many benefits of fiber, it's mind-boggling that the vast majority of people consume just half of the recommended amount. Fiber makes you feel full after meals, which makes it easier to fend off second helpings or a late-night snack attack. If you are cutting calories, it's easy to never quite feel full, so make fiber your go-to! Adequate fiber intake can help lower cholesterol, as well as prevent constipation and diverticulosis. And new research suggests that a healthy digestive tract contributes to appetite control. Fiber also plays a role in blunting blood sugar spikes and valleys, keeping blood sugar within a healthy range and avoiding the need for a quick sugar fix. Experts agree that every 1,000 calories consumed should be accompanied by 14 grams of fiber, and research has found that by simply focusing on an intake of 30 grams a day, dieters lost 5 pounds over a year. This week, make it your goal to include fiber in most eating occasions and strive to hit 30 grams every day.

FOOD	CAL	CARBS (G)	FIBER (G)	PROT (G)	FAT (G)	OTHER

Hunger ☒ ⊟ ☑ Mood ☒ ⊟ ☑

Hunger ☒ ⊟ ☑ Mood ☒ ⊟ ☑

Hunger ☒ ⊟ ☑ Mood ☒ ⊟ ☑

Hunger ☒ ⊟ ☑ Mood ☒ ⊟ ☑

DAILY TOTALS (G)

MACROS (%)

43

Fitness

Duration

Burn

Reflection

Fuel

Fluid ← ↔ →

Fuel ← ↔ →

Other ← ↔ →

FOOD	CAL	CARBS (G)	FIBER (G)	PROT (G)	FAT (G)	OTHER

Hunger ☒ ⊟ ☑   Mood ☒ ⊟ ☑

Hunger ☒ ⊟ ☑   Mood ☒ ⊟ ☑

Hunger ☒ ⊟ ☑   Mood ☒ ⊟ ☑

Hunger ☒ ⊟ ☑   Mood ☒ ⊟ ☑

DAILY TOTALS (G)

MACROS (%)

44

Fitness

Duration

Burn

Reflection

Fuel

Fluid ← ↔ →

Fuel ← ↔ →

Other ← ↔ →

FOOD	CAL	CARBS (G)	FIBER (G)	PROT (G)	FAT (G)	OTHER

Hunger ☒ ☐ ☑   Mood ☒ ☐ ☑

Hunger ☒ ☐ ☑   Mood ☒ ☐ ☑

Hunger ☒ ☐ ☑   Mood ☒ ☐ ☑

Hunger ☒ ☐ ☑   Mood ☒ ☐ ☑

DAILY TOTALS (G)

MACROS (%)

45

Fitness

Duration

Burn

Reflection

Fuel

Fluid ← ↔ →

Fuel ← ↔ →

Other ← ↔ →

FULLER, LONGER

FOOD	CAL	CARBS (G)	FIBER (G)	PROT (G)	FAT (G)	OTHER

Hunger ☒ ☐ ☑   Mood ☒ ☐ ☑

Hunger ☒ ☐ ☑   Mood ☒ ☐ ☑

Hunger ☒ ☐ ☑   Mood ☒ ☐ ☑

Hunger ☒ ☐ ☑   Mood ☒ ☐ ☑

DAILY TOTALS (G)

MACROS (%)

46

Fitness

Duration

Burn

Reflection

Fuel

Fluid ← ↔ →

Fuel ← ↔ →

Other ← ↔ →

FOOD	CAL	CARBS (G)	FIBER (G)	PROT (G)	FAT (G)	OTHER

Hunger ⊠ – ✓　Mood ⊠ – ✓

Hunger ⊠ – ✓　Mood ⊠ – ✓

Hunger ⊠ – ✓　Mood ⊠ – ✓

Hunger ⊠ – ✓　Mood ⊠ – ✓

DAILY TOTALS (G)

MACROS (%)

47

Fitness

Duration

Burn

Reflection

Fuel

Fluid　← ↔ →

Fuel　← ↔ →

Other　← ↔ →

FULLER, LONGER

FOOD	CAL	CARBS (G)	FIBER (G)	PROT (G)	FAT (G)	OTHER

Hunger ☒ ☐ ☑   Mood ☒ ☐ ☑

Hunger ☒ ☐ ☑   Mood ☒ ☐ ☑

Hunger ☒ ☐ ☑   Mood ☒ ☐ ☑

Hunger ☒ ☐ ☑   Mood ☒ ☐ ☑

DAILY TOTALS (G)

MACROS (%)

48

Fitness

Duration

Burn

Reflection

Fuel

Fluid ← ↔ →

Fuel ← ↔ →

Other ← ↔ →

FOOD	CAL	CARBS (G)	FIBER (G)	PROT (G)	FAT (G)	OTHER

Hunger ⊠ ─ ☑   Mood ⊠ ─ ☑

Hunger ⊠ ─ ☑   Mood ⊠ ─ ☑

Hunger ⊠ ─ ☑   Mood ⊠ ─ ☑

Hunger ⊠ ─ ☑   Mood ⊠ ─ ☑

DAILY TOTALS (G)

MACROS (%)

49

Fitness

Duration

Burn

Reflection

Fuel

Fluid ← ↔ →

Fuel ← ↔ →

Other ← ↔ →

FULLER, LONGER

Week 7 Review

Average weekly blend

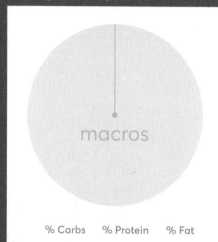

macros

% Carbs   % Protein   % Fat

Wins & losses

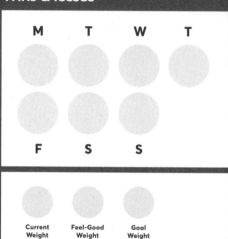

M   T   W   T

F   S   S

Current   Feel-Good   Goal
Weight   Weight   Weight

For a better tomorrow

Fitness   ☒ ☐ ☑

Next week I will . . .

Fuel   ☒ ☐ ☑

Next week I will . . .

Week 8

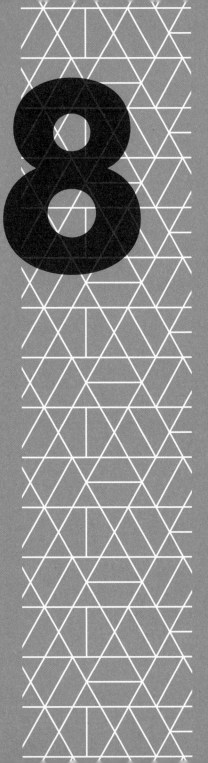

Believe in the power of protein

In the journey to get lean and toned, we need to shed fat while preserving muscle. But rapid weight loss often results in the loss of the muscle (you want to keep) along with the loss of fat (which you want to shed). In a recent study published in the *FASEB Journal*, dieters who consumed twice the recommended value for protein (or approximately 0.7 g/lb. of body weight) while cutting calories and exercising lost more fat yet preserved more lean muscle than those who stuck with the RDA alone. Protein plays a wide range of critical roles in the body, including the ability to protect lean body mass and satiate appetite, which leads to that lean, toned look. Eating small amounts of protein throughout the day—15+ grams per sitting, 4 to 6 times a day—helps to continuously protect and fuel muscles, satiate appetite, and fulfill the host of biological roles for which protein is essential. This week aim to consume a source of protein at each eating occasion, and extra accolades for you if you hit the 15+ gram goal per occasion!

FOOD	CAL	CARBS (G)	FIBER (G)	PROT (G)	FAT (G)	OTHER

Hunger ☒ ☐ ☑ Mood ☒ ☐ ☑

Hunger ☒ ☐ ☑ Mood ☒ ☐ ☑

Hunger ☒ ☐ ☑ Mood ☒ ☐ ☑

Hunger ☒ ☐ ☑ Mood ☒ ☐ ☑

DAILY TOTALS (G)

MACROS (%)

50

Fitness

Duration

Burn

Reflection

Fuel

Fluid ← ↔ →

Fuel ← ↔ →

Other ← ↔ →

FOOD		CAL	CARBS (G)	FIBER (G)	PROT (G)	FAT (G)	OTHER
					Hunger ☒ ☐ ☑		Mood ☒ ☐ ☑
					Hunger ☒ ☐ ☑		Mood ☒ ☐ ☑
					Hunger ☒ ☐ ☑		Mood ☒ ☐ ☑
					Hunger ☒ ☐ ☑		Mood ☒ ☐ ☑
DAILY TOTALS (G)							
MACROS (%)							

51

Fitness

Duration

Burn

Reflection

Fuel

Fluid ← ↔ →

Fuel ← ↔ →

Other ← ↔ →

FOOD	CAL	CARBS (G)	FIBER (G)	PROT (G)	FAT (G)	OTHER

Hunger ☒ ☐ ☑   Mood ☒ ☐ ☑

Hunger ☒ ☐ ☑   Mood ☒ ☐ ☑

Hunger ☒ ☐ ☑   Mood ☒ ☐ ☑

Hunger ☒ ☐ ☑   Mood ☒ ☐ ☑

DAILY TOTALS (G)

MACROS (%)

52

Fitness

Duration

Burn

Reflection

Fuel

Fluid ← ↔ →

Fuel ← ↔ →

Other ← ↔ →

FOOD	CAL	CARBS (G)	FIBER (G)	PROT (G)	FAT (G)	OTHER

Hunger ☒ ⊟ ☑   Mood ☒ ⊟ ☑

Hunger ☒ ⊟ ☑   Mood ☒ ⊟ ☑

Hunger ☒ ⊟ ☑   Mood ☒ ⊟ ☑

Hunger ☒ ⊟ ☑   Mood ☒ ⊟ ☑

DAILY TOTALS (G)

MACROS (%)

53

Fitness

Duration

Burn

Reflection

Fuel

Fluid   ← ↔ →

Fuel   ← ↔ →

Other   ← ↔ →

STRONGER, LONGER

FOOD	CAL	CARBS (G)	FIBER (G)	PROT (G)	FAT (G)	OTHER

Hunger ☒ ☐ ☑ Mood ☒ ☐ ☑

Hunger ☒ ☐ ☑ Mood ☒ ☐ ☑

Hunger ☒ ☐ ☑ Mood ☒ ☐ ☑

Hunger ☒ ☐ ☑ Mood ☒ ☐ ☑

DAILY TOTALS (G)

MACROS (%)

54

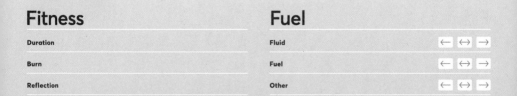

Fitness

Duration

Burn

Reflection

Fuel

Fluid ← ↔ →

Fuel ← ↔ →

Other ← ↔ →

FOOD	CAL	CARBS (G)	FIBER (G)	PROT (G)	FAT (G)	OTHER

Hunger ☒ ☐ ✓ Mood ☒ ☐ ✓

Hunger ☒ ☐ ✓ Mood ☒ ☐ ✓

Hunger ☒ ☐ ✓ Mood ☒ ☐ ✓

Hunger ☒ ☐ ✓ Mood ☒ ☐ ✓

DAILY TOTALS (G)

MACROS (%)

55

Fitness

Duration

Burn

Reflection

Fuel

Fluid ← ↔ →

Fuel ← ↔ →

Other ← ↔ →

STRONGER, LONGER

FOOD		CAL	CARBS (G)	FIBER (G)	PROT (G)	FAT (G)	OTHER
		Hunger ☒ ☐ ☑			Mood ☒ ☐ ☑		
		Hunger ☒ ☐ ☑			Mood ☒ ☐ ☑		
		Hunger ☒ ☐ ☑			Mood ☒ ☐ ☑		
		Hunger ☒ ☐ ☑			Mood ☒ ☐ ☑		

DAILY TOTALS (G)

MACROS (%)

Fitness

Duration

Burn

Reflection

Fuel

Fluid ← ↔ →

Fuel ← ↔ →

Other ← ↔ →

Week 8 Review

Average weekly blend

macros

% Carbs   % Protein   % Fat

Wins & losses

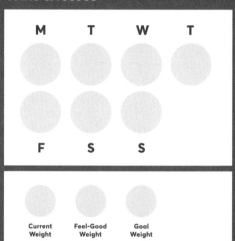

M	T	W	T
F	S	S	

Current Weight   Feel-Good Weight   Goal Weight

For a better tomorrow

Fitness ☒ ☐ ☑

Next week I will . . .

⇧

⇨

Fuel ☒ ☐ ☑

Next week I will . . .

⇧

⇨

Monthly Habit Tracker

No doubt there are some habits you want to make and others you want to break. Put them here and track your progress daily over the coming month.

	1	2	3	4	5	6	7	8	9	10	11	12	13	14	15	16
	17	18	19	20	21	22	23	24	25	26	27	28	29	30	31	

	1	2	3	4	5	6	7	8	9	10	11	12	13	14	15	16
	17	18	19	20	21	22	23	24	25	26	27	28	29	30	31	

	1	2	3	4	5	6	7	8	9	10	11	12	13	14	15	16
	17	18	19	20	21	22	23	24	25	26	27	28	29	30	31	

	1	2	3	4	5	6	7	8	9	10	11	12	13	14	15	16
	17	18	19	20	21	22	23	24	25	26	27	28	29	30	31	

	1	2	3	4	5	6	7	8	9	10	11	12	13	14	15	16
	17	18	19	20	21	22	23	24	25	26	27	28	29	30	31	

Week

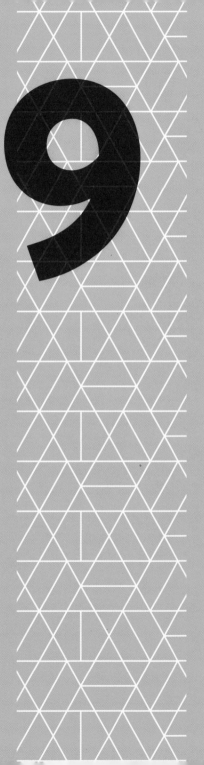

9

Focus on fitness

When looking at the scales of weight loss, there are two sides to the equation. *Calories in* stems from all of the food choices made throughout the day, the total volume of what's consumed. While there's generally more room for improvement there, when it comes to overall health and performance, it's more a question of calories out. *Calories out* stems from energy expended in the activities of daily living and from time spent sweating. This side of the equation impacts more than just your waistline and the number on the scale. If you're looking for wellness and longevity, don't quit your fitness habit! Fitness is king, and this week, make it your goal to do more than last week. If you worked out four days last week, let's make it five. If your previous workouts were light and short, let's pick up the pace or duration. Challenge yourself. I promise you that the benefits and euphoria of exercise far outweigh the effort.

FOOD	CAL	CARBS (G)	FIBER (G)	PROT (G)	FAT (G)	OTHER

Hunger ⊠ − √   Mood ⊠ − √

Hunger ⊠ − √   Mood ⊠ − √

Hunger ⊠ − √   Mood ⊠ − √

Hunger ⊠ − √   Mood ⊠ − √

DAILY TOTALS (G)

MACROS (%)

57

Fitness

Duration

Burn

Reflection

Fuel

Fluid ← ↔ →

Fuel ← ↔ →

Other ← ↔ →

FOOD		CAL	CARBS (G)	FIBER (G)	PROT (G)	FAT (G)	OTHER

Hunger × — √   Mood × — √

Hunger × — √   Mood × — √

Hunger × — √   Mood × — √

Hunger × — √   Mood × — √

DAILY TOTALS (G)

MACROS (%)

58

Fitness

Duration

Burn

Reflection

Fuel

Fluid   ← ↔ →

Fuel   ← ↔ →

Other   ← ↔ →

MOVE MORE

FOOD	CAL	CARBS (G)	FIBER (G)	PROT (G)	FAT (G)	OTHER

Hunger ☒ ☐ ☑   Mood ☒ ☐ ☑

Hunger ☒ ☐ ☑   Mood ☒ ☐ ☑

Hunger ☒ ☐ ☑   Mood ☒ ☐ ☑

Hunger ☒ ☐ ☑   Mood ☒ ☐ ☑

DAILY TOTALS (G)

MACROS (%)

59

Fitness

Duration

Burn

Reflection

Fuel

Fluid ← ↔ →

Fuel ← ↔ →

Other ← ↔ →

FOOD	CAL	CARBS (G)	FIBER (G)	PROT (G)	FAT (G)	OTHER
Hunger ☒ ☐ ☑ Mood ☒ ☐ ☑						
Hunger ☒ ☐ ☑ Mood ☒ ☐ ☑						
Hunger ☒ ☐ ☑ Mood ☒ ☐ ☑						
Hunger ☒ ☐ ☑ Mood ☒ ☐ ☑						
DAILY TOTALS (G)						
MACROS (%)						

60

Fitness

Duration

Burn

Reflection

Fuel

Fluid ← ↔ →

Fuel ← ↔ →

Other ← ↔ →

MOVE MORE

FOOD		CAL	CARBS (G)	FIBER (G)	PROT (G)	FAT (G)	OTHER

Hunger ☒ ☐ ☑ Mood ☒ ☐ ☑

Hunger ☒ ☐ ☑ Mood ☒ ☐ ☑

Hunger ☒ ☐ ☑ Mood ☒ ☐ ☑

Hunger ☒ ☐ ☑ Mood ☒ ☐ ☑

DAILY TOTALS (G)

MACROS (%)

61

Fitness

Duration

Burn

Reflection

Fuel

Fluid ← ↔ →

Fuel ← ↔ →

Other ← ↔ →

FOOD	CAL	CARBS (G)	FIBER (G)	PROT (G)	FAT (G)	OTHER

Hunger ⊠ ⊟ ☑   Mood ⊠ ⊟ ☑

Hunger ⊠ ⊟ ☑   Mood ⊠ ⊟ ☑

Hunger ⊠ ⊟ ☑   Mood ⊠ ⊟ ☑

Hunger ⊠ ⊟ ☑   Mood ⊠ ⊟ ☑

DAILY TOTALS (G)

MACROS (%)

62

Fitness

Duration

Burn

Reflection

Fuel

Fluid ← ↔ →

Fuel ← ↔ →

Other ← ↔ →

MOVE MORE

FOOD	CAL	CARBS (G)	FIBER (G)	PROT (G)	FAT (G)	OTHER

Hunger ☒ ☐ ☑   Mood ☒ ☐ ☑

Hunger ☒ ☐ ☑   Mood ☒ ☐ ☑

Hunger ☒ ☐ ☑   Mood ☒ ☐ ☑

Hunger ☒ ☐ ☑   Mood ☒ ☐ ☑

DAILY TOTALS (G)

MACROS (%)

63

Fitness

Duration

Burn

Reflection

Fuel

Fluid   ← ↔ →

Fuel   ← ↔ →

Other   ← ↔ →

Average weekly blend

macros

% Carbs   % Protein   % Fat

Wins & losses

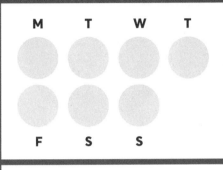

M   T   W   T

F   S   S

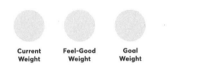

Current
Weight

Feel-Good
Weight

Goal
Weight

For a better tomorrow

Fitness   ☒ ⊟ ☑

⇧

Next week I will . . .

⇨

Fuel   ☒ ⊟ ☑

⇧

Next week I will . . .

⇨

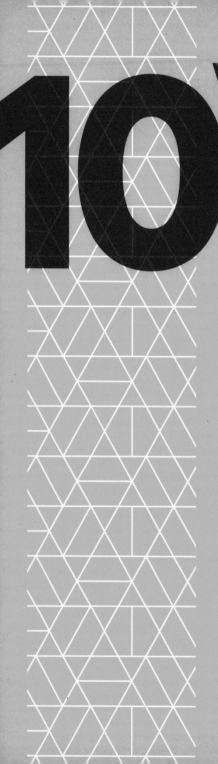

Week 10

Portions matter

There are many foods you can keep eating once you can get the portions right. But portion control can be confusing; a teaspoon of this, a half-cup of that, and pretty soon the fun of food prep is lost as you struggle to measure foods at each meal. This week try using visual cues to estimate those portion sizes; use your palm to "measure" proteins, your fist to "measure" carbs, and your thumb to "measure" fats. Aim for a blend of portions: carbs, protein, and fat at every meal so you consume energy that keeps you steady and satiated for hours to come. When you get portion fatigue, reach for vegetables. Only 1 in 10 adults consumes enough, and I guarantee you that expanding portions of nonstarchy veggies are not to blame for expanding waistlines! So give greens the green light and eat up!

FOOD	CAL	CARBS (G)	FIBER (G)	PROT (G)	FAT (G)	OTHER

Hunger ☒ ☐ ☑   Mood ☒ ☐ ☑

Hunger ☒ ☐ ☑   Mood ☒ ☐ ☑

Hunger ☒ ☐ ☑   Mood ☒ ☐ ☑

Hunger ☒ ☐ ☑   Mood ☒ ☐ ☑

DAILY TOTALS (G)

MACROS (%)

64

Fitness

Duration

Burn

Reflection

Fuel

Fluid   ← ↔ →

Fuel   ← ↔ →

Other   ← ↔ →

PORTIONS ON PURPOSE

FOOD							CAL	CARBS (G)	FIBER (G)	PROT (G)	FAT (G)	OTHER

Hunger ☒ ☐ ☑ Mood ☒ ☐ ☑

Hunger ☒ ☐ ☑ Mood ☒ ☐ ☑

Hunger ☒ ☐ ☑ Mood ☒ ☐ ☑

Hunger ☒ ☐ ☑ Mood ☒ ☐ ☑

DAILY TOTALS (G)

MACROS (%)

65

Fitness

Duration

Burn

Reflection

Fuel

Fluid ← ↔ →

Fuel ← ↔ →

Other ← ↔ →

FOOD		CAL	CARBS (G)	FIBER (G)	PROT (G)	FAT (G)	OTHER

Hunger ☒ ☐— ☐✓   Mood ☒ ☐— ☐✓

Hunger ☒ ☐— ☐✓   Mood ☒ ☐— ☐✓

Hunger ☒ ☐— ☐✓   Mood ☒ ☐— ☐✓

Hunger ☒ ☐— ☐✓   Mood ☒ ☐— ☐✓

DAILY TOTALS (G)

MACROS (%)

66

Fitness

Duration

Burn

Reflection

Fuel

Fluid ← ↔ →

Fuel ← ↔ →

Other ← ↔ →

FOOD	CAL	CARBS (G)	FIBER (G)	PROT (G)	FAT (G)	OTHER

Hunger ☒ ☐ ☑   Mood ☒ ☐ ☑

Hunger ☒ ☐ ☑   Mood ☒ ☐ ☑

Hunger ☒ ☐ ☑   Mood ☒ ☐ ☑

Hunger ☒ ☐ ☑   Mood ☒ ☐ ☑

DAILY TOTALS (G)

MACROS (%)

67

Fitness

Duration

Burn

Reflection

Fuel

Fluid   ← ↔ →

Fuel   ← ↔ →

Other   ← ↔ →

FOOD	CAL	CARBS (G)	FIBER (G)	PROT (G)	FAT (G)	OTHER

Hunger ☒ ☐ ☑   Mood ☒ ☐ ☑

Hunger ☒ ☐ ☑   Mood ☒ ☐ ☑

Hunger ☒ ☐ ☑   Mood ☒ ☐ ☑

Hunger ☒ ☐ ☑   Mood ☒ ☐ ☑

DAILY TOTALS (G)

MACROS (%)

68

Fitness

Duration

Burn

Reflection

Fuel

Fluid ← ↔ →

Fuel ← ↔ →

Other ← ↔ →

FOOD	CAL	CARBS (G)	FIBER (G)	PROT (G)	FAT (G)	OTHER

Hunger ☒ ☐ ☑   Mood ☒ ☐ ☑

Hunger ☒ ☐ ☑   Mood ☒ ☐ ☑

Hunger ☒ ☐ ☑   Mood ☒ ☐ ☑

Hunger ☒ ☐ ☑   Mood ☒ ☐ ☑

DAILY TOTALS (G)

MACROS (%)

69

Fitness

Duration

Burn

Reflection

Fuel

Fluid   ← ↔ →

Fuel   ← ↔ →

Other   ← ↔ →

FOOD		CAL	CARBS (G)	FIBER (G)	PROT (G)	FAT (G)	OTHER

Hunger ☒ ☐ ☑   Mood ☒ ☐ ☑

Hunger ☒ ☐ ☑   Mood ☒ ☐ ☑

Hunger ☒ ☐ ☑   Mood ☒ ☐ ☑

Hunger ☒ ☐ ☑   Mood ☒ ☐ ☑

DAILY TOTALS (G)

MACROS (%)

70

Fitness

Duration

Burn

Reflection

Fuel

Fluid   ← ↔ →

Fuel   ← ↔ →

Other   ← ↔ →

Week 10 Review

Average weekly blend

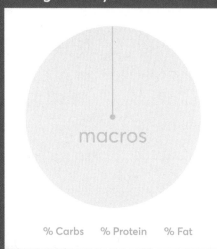

macros

% Carbs   % Protein   % Fat

Wins & losses

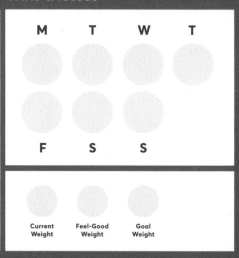

M   T   W   T

F   S   S

Current   Feel-Good   Goal
Weight   Weight   Weight

For a better tomorrow

Fitness   ☒ ☐ ☑

Next week I will . . .

Fuel   ☒ ☐ ☑

Next week I will . . .

Week
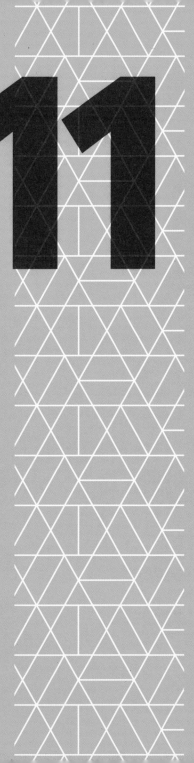

11

Don't go
it alone

As you near the end of your 90 days, it's time
to begin thinking about how you turn healthy
living into an everyday habit. Check in with
your support system. Stay in touch with friends
who encourage, check in, and make sure you
roll out of bed for that 6:00 a.m. workout.
Track down an expert who has spent years
providing prescriptive nutrition advice, life
hacks, and recipes to keep you intrigued.
Find a friend who can guide you around the
gym and the kitchen and who can make
exercise and cooking something you'll look
forward to. You'll need a stalwart guide who
will keep you in line, motivate you when
needed, hug you when you're discouraged,
high-five you when you succeed, and show
you by example that it's possible to be
mentally strong in a world full of donuts.

FOOD	CAL	CARBS (G)	FIBER (G)	PROT (G)	FAT (G)	OTHER

Hunger ☒ ☐ ☑ Mood ☒ ☐ ☑

Hunger ☒ ☐ ☑ Mood ☒ ☐ ☑

Hunger ☒ ☐ ☑ Mood ☒ ☐ ☑

Hunger ☒ ☐ ☑ Mood ☒ ☐ ☑

DAILY TOTALS (G)

MACROS (%)

71

Fitness

Duration

Burn

Reflection

Fuel

Fluid ← ↔ →

Fuel ← ↔ →

Other ← ↔ →

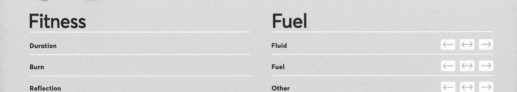

FOOD		CAL	CARBS (G)	FIBER (G)	PROT (G)	FAT (G)	OTHER
				Hunger ☒ ☐ ✓		Mood ☒ ☐ ✓	
				Hunger ☒ ☐ ✓		Mood ☒ ☐ ✓	
				Hunger ☒ ☐ ✓		Mood ☒ ☐ ✓	
				Hunger ☒ ☐ ✓		Mood ☒ ☐ ✓	
DAILY TOTALS (G)							
MACROS (%)							

72

Fitness

Duration

Burn

Reflection

Fuel

Fluid ← ↔ →

Fuel ← ↔ →

Other ← ↔ →

FIND YOUR CREW

FOOD		CAL	CARBS (G)	FIBER (G)	PROT (G)	FAT (G)	OTHER

Hunger ☒ ☐ ☑ Mood ☒ ☐ ☑

Hunger ☒ ☐ ☑ Mood ☒ ☐ ☑

Hunger ☒ ☐ ☑ Mood ☒ ☐ ☑

Hunger ☒ ☐ ☑ Mood ☒ ☐ ☑

DAILY TOTALS (G)

MACROS (%)

73

Fitness

Duration

Burn

Reflection

Fuel

Fluid ← ↔ →

Fuel ← ↔ →

Other ← ↔ →

FOOD	CAL	CARBS (G)	FIBER (G)	PROT (G)	FAT (G)	OTHER

Hunger ☒ ⊟ ☑   Mood ☒ ⊟ ☑

Hunger ☒ ⊟ ☑   Mood ☒ ⊟ ☑

Hunger ☒ ⊟ ☑   Mood ☒ ⊟ ☑

Hunger ☒ ⊟ ☑   Mood ☒ ⊟ ☑

DAILY TOTALS (G)

MACROS (%)

74

Fitness

Duration

Burn

Reflection

Fuel

Fluid ← ↔ →

Fuel ← ↔ →

Other ← ↔ →

FIND YOUR CREW

FOOD	CAL	CARBS (G)	FIBER (G)	PROT (G)	FAT (G)	OTHER

Hunger ☒ ☐ ☑   Mood ☒ ☐ ☑

Hunger ☒ ☐ ☑   Mood ☒ ☐ ☑

Hunger ☒ ☐ ☑   Mood ☒ ☐ ☑

Hunger ☒ ☐ ☑   Mood ☒ ☐ ☑

DAILY TOTALS (G)

MACROS (%)

75

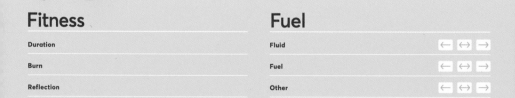

Fitness

Duration

Burn

Reflection

Fuel

Fluid   ← ↔ →

Fuel   ← ↔ →

Other   ← ↔ →

FOOD	CAL	CARBS (G)	FIBER (G)	PROT (G)	FAT (G)	OTHER

Hunger ☒ ☐ ☑   Mood ☒ ☐ ☑

Hunger ☒ ☐ ☑   Mood ☒ ☐ ☑

Hunger ☒ ☐ ☑   Mood ☒ ☐ ☑

Hunger ☒ ☐ ☑   Mood ☒ ☐ ☑

DAILY TOTALS (G)

MACROS (%)

76

Fitness

Duration

Burn

Reflection

Fuel

Fluid ← ↔ →

Fuel ← ↔ →

Other ← ↔ →

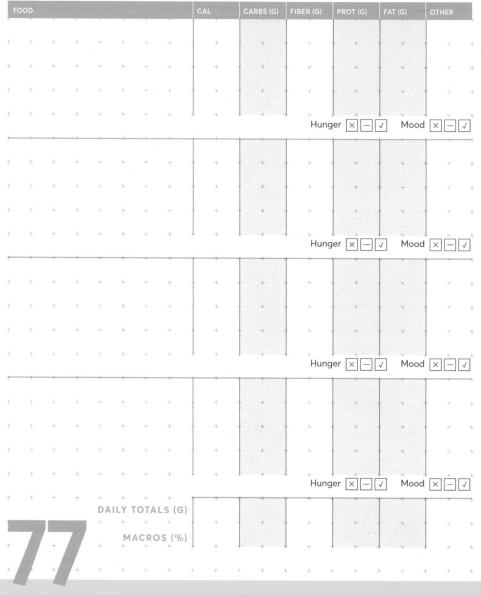

FOOD	CAL	CARBS (G)	FIBER (G)	PROT (G)	FAT (G)	OTHER

Hunger × — √   Mood × — √

Hunger × — √   Mood × — √

Hunger × — √   Mood × — √

Hunger × — √   Mood × — √

DAILY TOTALS (G)

MACROS (%)

77

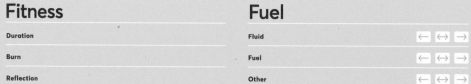

Fitness

Duration

Burn

Reflection

Fuel

Fluid ← ↔ →

Fuel ← ↔ →

Other ← ↔ →

Week 11 Review

Average weekly blend

macros

% Carbs   % Protein   % Fat

Wins & losses

M	T	W	T

F	S	S

Current Weight   Feel-Good Weight   Goal Weight

For a better tomorrow

Fitness   ☒ ⊟ ☑

Next week I will . . .

Fuel   ☒ ⊟ ☑

Next week I will . . .

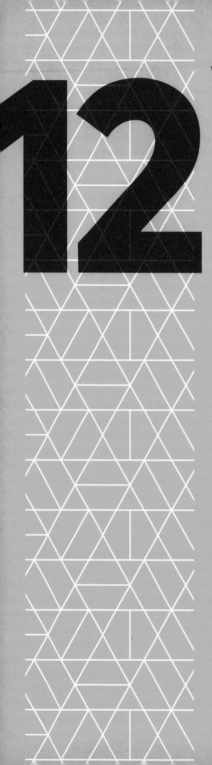

12

Week

Look long-term

Stay the course. Eating better and establishing a better relationship with food is a journey—complete with detours and setbacks—but the final destination offers beautiful views of better health and wellness. Whether you are on the hunt to find your ideal body weight and BMI or looking for continual progress along the path toward better numbers, reaching your healthy weight leads to a reduction in comorbidities and better whole health outcomes. And after weeks of this journey, you know that it takes work. There's no magic answer, no overnight success stories here. This week, revisit the list of essential foods (pp. 42–52) and make sure that your plate contains plenty of these nutrient-dense gems throughout the week. If you've made drastic body composition and weight changes, revisit the section on calculating energy needs (p. 66) and get updated on what your body needs now. And don't skip the section on sleep, stress, and support as these three things are critical to long-term success in eating and in health.

FOOD		CAL	CARBS (G)	FIBER (G)	PROT (G)	FAT (G)	OTHER
			Hunger ☒ — ☑		Mood ☒ — ☑		
			Hunger ☒ — ☑		Mood ☒ — ☑		
			Hunger ☒ — ☑		Mood ☒ — ☑		
			Hunger ☒ — ☑		Mood ☒ — ☑		
DAILY TOTALS (G)							
MACROS (%)							

78

Fitness

Duration

Burn

Reflection

Fuel

Fluid ← ↔ →

Fuel ← ↔ →

Other ← ↔ →

EYE ON THE PRIZE

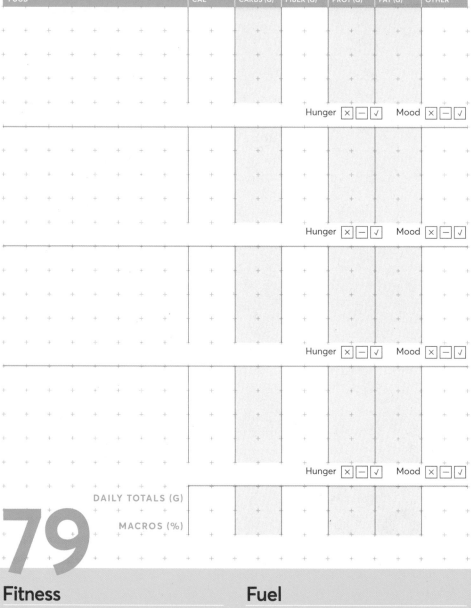

FOOD		CAL	CARBS (G)	FIBER (G)	PROT (G)	FAT (G)	OTHER

Hunger ☒ ☐ ☑ Mood ☒ ☐ ☑

Hunger ☒ ☐ ☑ Mood ☒ ☐ ☑

Hunger ☒ ☐ ☑ Mood ☒ ☐ ☑

Hunger ☒ ☐ ☑ Mood ☒ ☐ ☑

DAILY TOTALS (G)

MACROS (%)

79

Fitness

Duration

Burn

Reflection

Fuel

Fluid ← ↔ →

Fuel ← ↔ →

Other ← ↔ →

FOOD	CAL	CARBS (G)	FIBER (G)	PROT (G)	FAT (G)	OTHER

Hunger ⊠ — ✓   Mood ⊠ — ✓

Hunger ⊠ — ✓   Mood ⊠ — ✓

Hunger ⊠ — ✓   Mood ⊠ — ✓

Hunger ⊠ — ✓   Mood ⊠ — ✓

DAILY TOTALS (G)

MACROS (%)

80

Fitness

Duration

Burn

Reflection

Fuel

Fluid ← ↔ →

Fuel ← ↔ →

Other ← ↔ →

EYE ON THE PRIZE

FOOD	CAL	CARBS (G)	FIBER (G)	PROT (G)	FAT (G)	OTHER

Hunger ☒ — ☑   Mood ☒ — ☑

Hunger ☒ — ☑   Mood ☒ — ☑

Hunger ☒ — ☑   Mood ☒ — ☑

Hunger ☒ — ☑   Mood ☒ — ☑

| DAILY TOTALS (G) | | | | | | |
| MACROS (%) | | | | | | |

81

Fitness

Duration

Burn

Reflection

Fuel

Fluid   ← ↔ →

Fuel   ← ↔ →

Other   ← ↔ →

FOOD	CAL	CARBS (G)	FIBER (G)	PROT (G)	FAT (G)	OTHER

Hunger ☒ ☐ ☑   Mood ☒ ☐ ☑

Hunger ☒ ☐ ☑   Mood ☒ ☐ ☑

Hunger ☒ ☐ ☑   Mood ☒ ☐ ☑

Hunger ☒ ☐ ☑   Mood ☒ ☐ ☑

DAILY TOTALS (G)

MACROS (%)

82

Fitness

Duration

Burn

Reflection

Fuel

Fluid ← ↔ →

Fuel ← ↔ →

Other ← ↔ →

EYE ON THE PRIZE

FOOD	CAL	CARBS (G)	FIBER (G)	PROT (G)	FAT (G)	OTHER

Hunger ☒ — ☑ Mood ☒ — ☑

Hunger ☒ — ☑ Mood ☒ — ☑

Hunger ☒ — ☑ Mood ☒ — ☑

Hunger ☒ — ☑ Mood ☒ — ☑

DAILY TOTALS (G)

MACROS (%)

83

Fitness

Duration

Burn

Reflection

Fuel

Fluid ← ↔ →

Fuel ← ↔ →

Other ← ↔ →

FOOD	CAL	CARBS (G)	FIBER (G)	PROT (G)	FAT (G)	OTHER

Hunger ☒ ☐ ☑   Mood ☒ ☐ ☑

Hunger ☒ ☐ ☑   Mood ☒ ☐ ☑

Hunger ☒ ☐ ☑   Mood ☒ ☐ ☑

Hunger ☒ ☐ ☑   Mood ☒ ☐ ☑

DAILY TOTALS (G)

MACROS (%)

84

Fitness

Duration

Burn

Reflection

Fuel

Fluid ← ↔ →

Fuel ← ↔ →

Other ← ↔ →

Week 12 Review

Average weekly blend

macros

% Carbs   % Protein   % Fat

Wins & losses

| M | T | W | T |
| F | S | S | |

Current Weight   Feel-Good Weight   Goal Weight

For a better tomorrow

Fitness   ☒ ☐ ☑

Next week I will . . .

Fuel   ☒ ☐ ☑

Next week I will . . .

Week 13

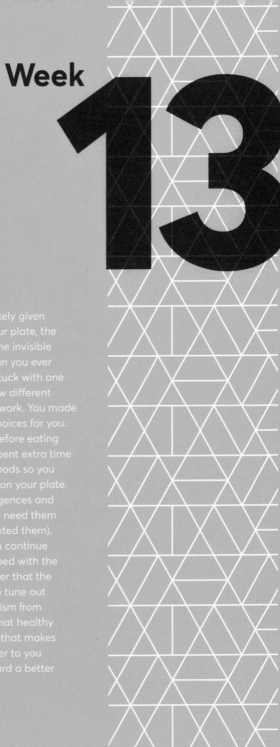

You are better today

Over the past 90 days, you've likely given more thought to the food on your plate, the nourishment in your belly, and the invisible factors that influence health than you ever have before. And whether you stuck with one plan throughout or tried on a few different diets for size, you put in a lot of work. You made it happen. No one made your choices for you. No one but you thought twice before eating certain foods. No one but you spent extra time measuring and portioning out foods so you could see what they looked like on your plate. No one but you said no to indulgences and added sugar because you didn't need them (even though you may have wanted them). You did the work here. So as you continue on your nutrition journey, equipped with the skills you have learned, remember that the choices you make, make you. So tune out the unsolicited advice and criticism from others and continue to pursue that healthy relationship with food, a weight that makes you happy, and goals that matter to you and continually inspire you toward a better tomorrow. You do you.

FOOD	CAL	CARBS (G)	FIBER (G)	PROT (G)	FAT (G)	OTHER

Hunger ☒ ☐ ☑ Mood ☒ ☐ ☑

Hunger ☒ ☐ ☑ Mood ☒ ☐ ☑

Hunger ☒ ☐ ☑ Mood ☒ ☐ ☑

Hunger ☒ ☐ ☑ Mood ☒ ☐ ☑

DAILY TOTALS (G)

MACROS (%)

85

Fitness

Duration

Burn

Reflection

Fuel

Fluid ← ↔ →

Fuel ← ↔ →

Other ← ↔ →

FOOD		CAL	CARBS (G)	FIBER (G)	PROT (G)	FAT (G)	OTHER
Hunger ☒ ☐ ☑ Mood ☒ ☐ ☑							
Hunger ☒ ☐ ☑ Mood ☒ ☐ ☑							
Hunger ☒ ☐ ☑ Mood ☒ ☐ ☑							
Hunger ☒ ☐ ☑ Mood ☒ ☐ ☑							
DAILY TOTALS (G)							
MACROS (%)							

86

Fitness

Duration

Burn

Reflection

Fuel

Fluid ← ↔ →

Fuel ← ↔ →

Other ← ↔ →

STAY STRONG, KEEP ON

FOOD	CAL	CARBS (G)	FIBER (G)	PROT (G)	FAT (G)	OTHER

Hunger ☒ ☐ ☑   Mood ☒ ☐ ☑

Hunger ☒ ☐ ☑   Mood ☒ ☐ ☑

Hunger ☒ ☐ ☑   Mood ☒ ☐ ☑

Hunger ☒ ☐ ☑   Mood ☒ ☐ ☑

DAILY TOTALS (G)

MACROS (%)

87

Fitness

Duration

Burn

Reflection

Fuel

Fluid ← ↔ →

Fuel ← ↔ →

Other ← ↔ →

FOOD	CAL	CARBS (G)	FIBER (G)	PROT (G)	FAT (G)	OTHER

Hunger ☒ ☐ ☑ Mood ☒ ☐ ☑

Hunger ☒ ☐ ☑ Mood ☒ ☐ ☑

Hunger ☒ ☐ ☑ Mood ☒ ☐ ☑

Hunger ☒ ☐ ☑ Mood ☒ ☐ ☑

DAILY TOTALS (G)

MACROS (%)

88

Fitness

Duration

Burn

Reflection

Fuel

Fluid ← ↔ →

Fuel ← ↔ →

Other ← ↔ →

FOOD	CAL	CARBS (G)	FIBER (G)	PROT (G)	FAT (G)	OTHER

Hunger ☒ ☐ ☑   Mood ☒ ☐ ☑

Hunger ☒ ☐ ☑   Mood ☒ ☐ ☑

Hunger ☒ ☐ ☑   Mood ☒ ☐ ☑

Hunger ☒ ☐ ☑   Mood ☒ ☐ ☑

DAILY TOTALS (G)

MACROS (%)

89

Fitness

Duration

Burn

Reflection

Fuel

Fluid ← ↔ →

Fuel ← ↔ →

Other ← ↔ →

FOOD		CAL	CARBS (G)	FIBER (G)	PROT (G)	FAT (G)	OTHER

Hunger ☒ ☐ ☑ Mood ☒ ☐ ☑

Hunger ☒ ☐ ☑ Mood ☒ ☐ ☑

Hunger ☒ ☐ ☑ Mood ☒ ☐ ☑

Hunger ☒ ☐ ☑ Mood ☒ ☐ ☑

DAILY TOTALS (G)

MACROS (%)

90

Fitness

Duration

Burn

Reflection

Fuel

Fluid ← ↔ →

Fuel ← ↔ →

Other ← ↔ →

STAY STRONG, KEEP ON

Week 13 Review

Average weekly blend

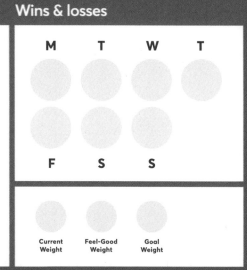

macros

% Carbs   % Protein   % Fat

Wins & losses

M	T	W	T

F	S	S

Current Weight   Feel-Good Weight   Goal Weight

For a better tomorrow

Fitness   ☒ ⊟ ☑

Next week I will . . .

⇧

⇨

Fuel   ☒ ⊟ ☑

Next week I will . . .

⇧

⇨

References

Part 1

Dirks, A. J., and C. Leeuwenburgh. "Caloric Restriction in Humans: Potential Pitfalls and Health Concerns." *Mechanisms of Aging and Development* 127, no. 1 (January 2006): 1–7. doi:10.1016/j.mad.2005.09.001

Ebbeling, C., et al. "Effects of a Low Carbohydrate Diet on Energy Expenditure During Weight Loss Maintenance: Randomized Trial." *BMJ* 363 (2018). www.bmj.com /content/363/bmj.k4583

Ganley, R. M. "Emotion and Eating in Obesity: A Review of the Literature." *International Journal of Eating Disorders* 8, no. 3 (1989): 343–361.

Harvie, M. N., M. Pegington, M. P. Mattson, J. Frystyk, B. Dillon, G. Evans, and J. Cuzick, et al. "The Effects of Intermittent or Continuous Energy Restriction on Weight Loss and Metabolic Disease Risk Markers: A Randomized Trial in Young Overweight Women." *International Journal of Obesity* 35, no. 5 (May 2011): 714–727. doi:10.1038/ijo.2010.171

Hawks, S. R., and J. Gast. "Weight Loss Management: A Path Lit Darkly." *Health Education & Behavior* 25, no. 3 (June 1998): 371–382. doi:10.1177/109019819802500310

Heilbronn, L. K., A. E. Civitarese, I. Bogacka, S. R. Smith, M. Hulver, and E. Ravussin. "Glucose Tolerance and Skeletal Muscle Gene Expression in Response to Alternate Day Fasting." *Obesity Research* 13, no. 3 (March 2005): 574–581. doi:10.1038/oby.2005.61

Heilbronn, L. K., S. R. Smith, C. K. Martin, S. D. Anton, and E. Ravussin. "Alternate-Day Fasting in Nonobese Subjects: Effects on Body Weight, Body Composition, and Energy Metabolism." *The American Journal of Clinical Nutrition* 81, no. 1 (January 2005): 69–73.

Johnstone, A. M. "Fasting—The Ultimate Diet?" *Obesity Reviews* 8, no. 3 (May 2007): 211–222. doi:10.1111/j.1467-789X.2006.00266.x

Kaushal, N., and R. E. Rhodes. "Exercise Habit Formation in New Gym Members: A Longitudinal Study." *Journal of Behavioral Medicine* 38, no. 4: 652–663.

Kerksick, C. M., et al. "International Society of Sports Nutrition Position Stand: Nutrient Timing." *Journal of the International Society of Sports Nutrition* 14, no. 1 (2017): 1–21. doi: 10.1186/s12970-017-0189-4

Laursen, P. B., and D. G. Jenkins. "The Scientific Basis for High-Intensity Interval Training: Optimising Training Programmes and Maximising Performance in Highly Trained Endurance Athletes." *Sports Medicine* (Auckland, NZ) 32, no. 1 (2002): 53–73.

Layman, D. K., et al. "A Reduced Ratio of Dietary Carbohydrate to Protein Improves Body Composition and Blood Lipid Profiles During Weight Loss in Adult Women." *Journal of Nutrition* 133 (2003): 411–417.

Longo, V. D., and M. P. Mattson. "Fasting: Molecular Mechanisms and Clinical Applications." *Cell Metabolism* 19, no. 2 (January 2014): 181–192. doi:10.1016/j.cmet.2013.12.008

Trepanokski, J., C. Kroeger, and A. Barnosky. "Effect of Alternate-Day Fasting on Weight Loss, Weight Maintenance, and Cardioprotection Among Metabocially Healthy Obese Adults." *JAMA Internal Medicine* 177, no. 7 (2017): 930–938. https://jamanetwork.com/journals/jamainternalmedicine/article-abstract/2623528

Varady, K. A. "Intermittent Versus Daily Calorie Restriction: Which Diet Regimen Is More Effective for Weight Loss?" *Obesity Reviews* 12, no. 7 (July 2011): e593–601. doi:10.1111/j.1467-789X.2011.00873.x

Varnier, M., P. Sarto, D. Martines, L. Lora, F. Carmignoto, G. P. Leese, and R. Naccarato. "Effect of Infusing Branched-Chain Amino Acid during Incremental Exercise with Reduced Muscle Glycogen Content." *European Journal of Applied Physiology* 69, no. 1 (1994): 26–31.

Part 2

American Dietetic Association. "Position of the Academy of Nutrition and Dietetics, Dietitians of Canada, and the American College of Sports Medicine: Nutrition and Athletic Performance." *Journal of the Academy of Nutrition and Dietetics* 116, no. 3 (2016): 501–528.

Burke, L. M., et al. "Guidelines for Daily Carbohydrate Intake: Do Athletes Achieve Them?" *Sports Medicine* 31, no. 4 (2001): 267–299.

Copinschi, G., R. Leproult, and K. Spiegel. "The Important Role of Sleep in Metabolism." *Frontiers of Hormone Research* 42 (2014): 5972. doi: 10.1159/000358858

Groesz, L., et al. "What Is Eating You? Stress and the Drive to Eat." *Appetite* 58, no. 2 (2012): 717–721.

Mifflin, M. D., et al. "A New Predictive Equation for Resting Energy Expenditure in Healthy Individuals." *The American Journal of Clinical Nutrition* 21, no. 2 (1990): 241–247. https://www.ncbi.nlm.nih.gov/pubmed/?term=Mifflin+%2C+predictive+equation+for+resting+energy+expen

Mumme, K., and W. Stonehouse. "Effects of Medium-Chain Triglycerides on Weight Loss and Body Composition: A Meta-Analysis of Randomized Controlled Trials." *Journal of the Academy of Nutrition and Dietetics* 115, no. 2 (2015): 249–263.

National Research Council. *Recommended Dietary Allowances*, 10th Ed. Washington DC: National Academy Press, 1989.

National Sleep Foundation. "Sleep and Effectiveness Are Linked, but Few Plan Their Sleep." https://www.sleepfoundation.org/sites/default/files/inline-files/Sleep%20in%20America%202018_prioritizing%20sleep_1.pdf

Patel, S. R., et al. "Association Between Reduced Sleep and Weight Gain in Women." *American Journal of Epidemiology* 164, no. 10 (November 2006): 947–954.

Patel, S. R., and F. Hu. "Short Sleep Duration and Weight Gain: A Systematic Review." *Obesity* 16, no. 3 (2008): 643–653.

Phillips, S. M., and L. J. Van Loon. "Dietary Protein for Athletes: From Requirements to Optimum Adaptation." *Journal of Sports Science* 19 (2011): S29–38. https://www.ncbi.nlm.nih.gov/pubmed/22150425

Rihm, J., et al. "Sleep Deprivation Selectively Upregulates an Amygdala–Hypothalamic Circuit Involved in Food Reward." *Journal of Neuroscience* 39, no. 5: 888–899.

Shirreffs, S. M., and M. N. Sawka. "Fluid and Electrolyte Needs for Training, Competition, and Recovery." *Journal of Sports Science* 29, Suppl 1 (2011): S39–46.

Taheri, S., L. Lin, D. Austin, T. Young, and E. Mignot. "Short Sleep Duration is Associated with Reduced Leptin, Elevated Ghrelin, and Increased Body Mass Index." *PLoS Medicine* 1, no. 3 (2004): e62. https://www.ncbi.nlm.nih.gov/pubmed/15602591

Wilson, J. M., et al. "The Effects of Ketogenic Dieting on Body Composition, Strength, Power, and Hormonal Profiles in Resistance Training Males." *The Journal of Strength and Conditioning Research* (2017) doi: 10.1519/JSC.0000000000001935

References

Acknowledgments

We know in life that no man, no woman, is an island. When I'm asked how I do it all, the answer is simple: I don't. I wrote this book with the help of family, friends, and experts. I was able to research and write late into the night because Jason Bede stepped up and kept our family functioning. And on weekends, Judy and Lou Bede and Mary and Stan Nisevich took my young kids to the park, loved on them, and kept them well-fed. My family benefitted from a rising tide of effort and passion while I pushed onward. *Sweat. Eat. Repeat.* came together thanks to Renee Jardine at VeloPress, and plenty of insights and advice from world-class athletes, dietitians, experts, and other all-around amazing human beings. Here's to the villages that support us.

I wrote this book for you, the reader. Whether you are working to quiet the call of junk food, trying to muster the motivation to break a sweat, or looking to reverse the habits you've created before you go mad, you can use this book to make meaningful, healthy changes in your life. I hope you find pearls of wisdom, plenty of acceptance, and some tough love, too. Let's read up and reflect and reach for something better together.

About the Author

As a marathoner, triathlete, registered dietitian, and certified specialist in sports dietetics, Pamela Nisevich Bede knows firsthand the important role nutrition plays in athletic performance, and in life itself. Having finished 23 marathons and an Ironman triathlon, and currently working to balance life as a working mom of three, Pamela offers reliable insight, gained through sweat equity and seeded in research. Pamela is known for passionately sharing expert nutrition advice with athletes, weight-loss warriors, general wellness seekers, and health professionals. She shares this expertise across media platforms and in person as owner of Swim, Bike, Run, Eat!, a private nutrition consulting firm.

A former collegiate soccer player turned endurance athlete, Pamela has authored or contributed to multiple books, including *Runner's World Big Book of Marathon and Half-Marathon Training*, *Runner's World Big Book of Running for Beginners*, *Runner's World Run to Lose*, and *Pocket Posh Dining Out Calorie Counter*. She writes for trade and consumer publications and is an open-minded expert, frequently quoted in publications such as *Triathlete*, *Men's Health*, *US News*, *More*, *Self*, *Huffington Post*, and *Runner's World* magazine.

Pamela's early roots are in education and clinical nutrition, where she worked as a pediatric clinical dietitian in the areas of inborn errors of metabolism, ketogenic diet for epilepsy, pediatric obesity, type 1 diabetes, and general pediatrics. When not writing or counseling clients,

Pamela works at a Fortune 500 company, where she focuses on nutrition science, external engagement, innovation, and educational content creation.

Pamela earned a bachelor of science degree in dietetics from Miami University and a master of science in medical dietetics from the Ohio State University. She enjoys nothing more than spending time with her three young children and husband, cooking and baking, and logging miles on her bike and in her running shoes.